Steel Love

By Deane Johnson

Text copyright ©2016 Deane Johnson
Cover illustration by J.R. Fleming
All rights reserved.
www.deaneandjoe.com

No part of this publication may be re-produced, stored in a retrieval system, or transmitted in any form or by any means, electronic, mechanical, photocopying, recording, or otherwise, without written permission of the publisher. For information regarding permission, contact Deane Johnson:

deanejohnson@twc.com

ISBN 978-1534812598

Dedicated to my husband, Judge Joe N. Johnson . . .
Father, Musician, X-Ray technician, Army veteran, TV Reporter,
Journalist, Justice Of The Peace, Lawyer, and District Judge.
We had 63 years and three months together on a Magic Carpet Ride.

*"It is not the strongest of the species that survives,
nor the most intelligent that survives.
It is the one that is most adaptable to change."
-Charles Darwin*

*"There is a sacredness in tears.
They are not the mark of weakness, but of power.
They speak more eloquently than ten-thousand tongues.
They are the messengers of overwhelming grief, of deep contrition,
and of unspeakable love."
-Washington Irving*

*Love conquers all.
-Virgil*

Contents

Foreword	p. 9
Introduction: Alzheimer's World	p. 11
2010	p. 19
2011	p. 41
2012	p. 59
2013	p. 73
2014	p. 87
2015	p. 109
Joe's Obituary	p. 125
Special Letters	p. 133
Acknowledgments	p. 141
Emails From Readers and Friends	p. 147

Foreword

The most beautiful aspect of a "suddenly" happens when you realize you were not looking for something to happen. Fortunately, our "suddenly" materialized through a beautiful relationship with one of the most interesting, candid, lusty, and transparently-charged individuals we've ever known. To experience all of those things with any one person is rare. To experience them with an octogenarian is priceless!

Within five minutes of being with Deane Johnson, you realize this is a woman who has lived some life. What she has been through has changed her for the good. Her respect for love has brought her to a place of being a brilliant voice of courage and hope for anyone who is facing his or her mountain. You want to talk about shadows? She's been there. You want to purge the pain from your loss? She'll understand your tears. You want to grieve the frustration of what sickness and death does to your loved one's life? She'll hold your hand and affirm to you the peace and comfort of God.

Deane writes as she feels, and she feels what she knows with full effect. You, the reader, will realize that you've been handed a gift as you crack into the vaults of Deane's memory and experience. She shares because she believes it will help.

Deane helped us, and she'll help you. Let her words help.

Oh, how we love this woman!

Mike & Patti Paschall
Authors of *Til Death Do Us Part*

Introduction:
Alzheimer's World

I have published another book called *I'll Be Seeing You*, which documents my husband's Alzheimer's from the time he was diagnosed in 2003 until we moved him into a care facility in 2010. It is available at www.amazon.com. I highly recommend reading that book before you begin this one, so that you can gain a fuller understanding of the Alzheimer's journey.

The book you currently hold in your hands, *Steel Love*, documents my husband's Alzheimer's from the time we moved him into the care facility in 2010 until his death in 2015. It is the other half of the story, thus a sequel. In the following pages, you will witness the final stages of this life-altering disease as well as the mental and physical decline of a man who was admired by all who knew him.

I now invite you to travel with me to the end of Joe's life. It was not an easy journey for me to take, but I hope my journal entries provide a glimpse into the daily trials of living with Alzheimer's. If you are going through a similar journey, please know that you are not alone.

-Deane Johnson

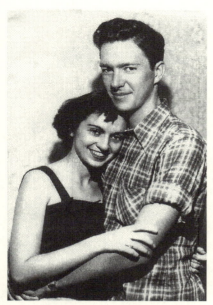

Joe and Deane, May 1951.

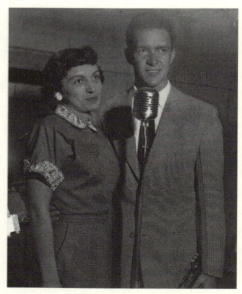

December 31, 1950. At Casa Blanca.
The night of our first kiss.

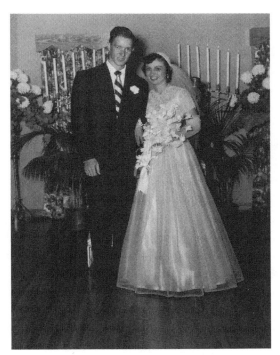

Joe and Deane's wedding day. October 27, 1951.

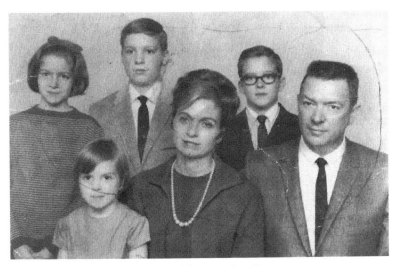

Back row: Mindy, Joe Jr., Barry
Front row: Dena, Deane, Joe

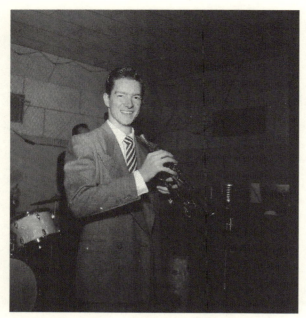

Joe with trumpet at Casa Blanca.

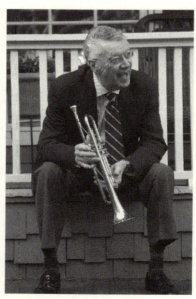

Joe with trumpet, 2005.

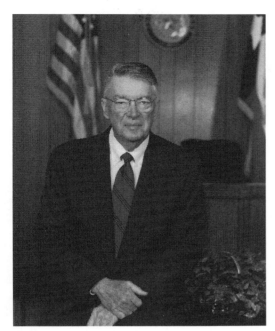

Joe as Judge of 170th District Court.

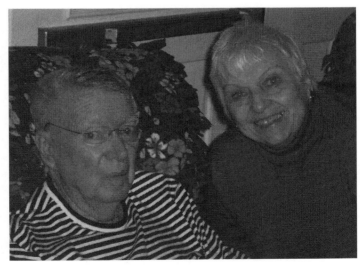

Joe and Deane at Sodalis, 2011.

16

The Journal
(2010-2015)

2010

Entry # 1

Another long day stares me in the face . . .

Something kept nudging me this afternoon, causing me to worry about Joe. I wanted to call him on the phone and chat with him for a while, but I decided it wasn't best. If he recognized my voice, he might worry about where I am and if I'm safe, or he will want to be with me. So instead, I called over to the facility—Sodalis—and asked how Joe was doing.

Arlene, a care worker, said Joe wouldn't come to the table at meal time because he was waiting for me to get there. Joe said he knew I must be hungry, and that he wanted to eat with me. So I went right over.

When I arrived about 5:30p.m., Joe was sitting in the den waiting for me so that we could go eat. After talking with him for a moment, I came to realize that he thought we were in Vegas. In his mind, I was up in our hotel room, and he was waiting on me in the lobby to meet him for dinner.

I was consoled, knowing that Joe, in his state of mind, was in a happy place. I stayed with him until 8p.m. It is always hard to leave him, because he thinks he is going home with me. He doesn't understand that the facility is his new home.

Needless to say, sadness abounds at every turn.

Entry #2

Jose Perez trimmed our trees this afternoon, and he asked me if I would sell him our 1993 navy Cadillac. Later, as I was watching TV, I was overcome with grief. I sat in my chair, crying in the dark, trying to figure out what brought forth the tears. Suddenly, it dawned on me. For years, whenever Perez trimmed the trees, Joe and I were outside together pointing out the limbs that we wanted him to cut. But today, I sat alone on the patio watching Perez trim the trees. The car was another incident that opened the flood gates. I couldn't sell the car. Joe found it for me 13 years ago. If that car left the car port, it would be like Joe leaving all over again. This is another piece of the grief puzzle.

Entry #3

After being overcome with sadness last night, I wanted to see Joe today. I bought us both Blizzards from Dairy Queen. We sat close together, hugged, stole a few kisses, and enjoyed our Blizzards. When dinner was served at 5p.m., I had tea. I started trying to leave about 7p.m., but it wasn't easy. I guess this is a preview of the rest of my life. I live in our house, and Joe lives in his home away from our home.

Entry #4

When a friend or family member accompanies me when I go visit Joe, it upsets him if we leave at the same time. But if we leave one at a time, Joe doesn't get upset.

Entry #5

Jackson and Eric, my twin grandsons, came over for a visit. While they were here, Sodalis called. Joe was sun downing. The twins took me right over to see him. We sat there for a short time, then I picked up on what Joe was thinking. Joe was holding court, and when he saw me he said I had no business at the court house. It's always been his belief that you don't take your wife with you to work.

So I got up, told him bye to make him believe that I was leaving, and went to the car to wait on the twins. Joe never thought family should come to work with him. In his sun downing mind, this was real, he was holding court, and when he saw me he wanted me out of his court room. Out I went. The boys stayed for a while. When they left, Joe was almost out of the zone.

Entry #6

My daughter, Mindy, and I went to see the movie *Sex in the City*. Joe would have enjoyed it. Then my son, Barry, and I had an enjoyable dinner at the Elite Café, and talked nonstop. Our children understand my loneliness and this solo journey I am now on. I confess that I often wonder if I will ever experience contentment again.

Entry #7

Jackson and Eric went with me to see Joe in order to celebrate my 80th birthday. I took a cake, and we enjoyed the celebration. Joe kept asking what the occasion was. There was a time when I would have reacted in a negative way to his question, but this disease has taught me to be less selfish. I didn't let it bother me, and enjoyed just being with Joe without any fanfare from him. I guess I'm growing up. Alzheimer's speeds up the maturing process. If it didn't, you would find me in my bed in a fetal position.

Later, we all met at the Elite with the Waco families minus Joe. It was hard for me to celebrate my birthday or any occasion without Joe, but I made it without crying. I am quieter than usual when I am with our families. I don't know why. I suppose it's because I am one from a marriage of two, and I am missing my other half.

Entry #8

I called over to Sodalis to check on Joe. He was at the dining table holding court. At that moment, in his mind, he was the judge in his court room. Charles, a visitor, stood up and put on his hat. It was then that Joe noticed Charles' wife was wearing shorts. When they got up to leave, he told them they had to leave because their attire was not acceptable in *his* court room. Joe never allowed anyone to wear a hat or shorts in his court room. The couple left immediately. It is amazing the way those suffering with Alzheimer's go back in time and remember the way things once were.

Entry #9

This month, we have taken Joe out to eat many times. I visited him at least four times a week or more. I want to see him every day, but each visit takes a lot out of me. The day after a visit, I always sit in my chair, tired and sad. It leaves me emotionally exhausted every time.

Entry #10

I have been having bad dreams. In every dream, I am struggling to make everything right. I wonder if Joe's and my living arrangements (i.e., living apart) are the cause of the dreams. Nights are nightmares of the reality in which I live.

Entry #11

Jimmy Johnson, our minister, came by to serve me communion. We had a nice visit. I am still sleeping long hours. I wonder if I will ever catch up on my sleep.

Entry #12

Thoughts of my children . . .

Jody calls me almost every day or every other day. Mindy is always available. Barry has his hands full every day making ends meet. Dena has her heart *and* hands full—Eric, Dena's husband, has been diagnosed with stage four throat cancer.

Life is full of unexpected trials.

Entry #13

In September, I visited Joe often. I slept late almost every day. I don't think I am that depressed, but I have never been this tired and this lonely before. Jackson and Eric help fill up my weeks. They bring their friends over, we go out to eat or splurge ourselves with a Blizzard. Looking back over my journal, I realize that I've been crying twelve days out of seventeen. Will my tears ever slow down? I don't see it happening.

Entry #14

Jody came for a visit, and we took Joe out to eat and for a ride around town. We dropped him off at Sodalis, and then Joe and I were separated again. I am forever grateful for the time our children spend with us. Their visits and phone calls are like a B-12 shot. Jody encouraged me to see my counselor, Mary Ann, regularly, and I do.

Entry #15

I had a surprise today. Karen Klaras Goss brought me a dozen yellow roses. Friends are priceless.

Entry #16

I have been dedicated to correcting my book, *I'll Be Seeing You*, for Jonathan. With any luck at all, I think this seven-year journal may be published. I hope it will help a lot of families on the Alzheimer's journey.

Entry #17

I took Joe's trumpet to Sodalis. When he saw his horn, he thought he had a band job he needed to get to immediately. He carried his horn into the backyard and tried to get out of the fenced yard to go play his gig.

One of the workers, Franscesca, wanted to hear Joe play, and he played for about an hour.

Entry #18

I feel bad saying that all my days are empty. Where do I find joy? Joe lives only three miles from me. I still find joy sitting close to him, stealing a kiss, and eating with him. But the time comes when I must find a way to leave without upsetting him and return to an empty house. I haven't been alone for over sixty years.

I don't remember the last day when I enjoyed a day from morning until bed time. Even though I was able to be close to Joe when he lived at home during the early stages of Alzheimer's, my days and evenings were spent on pins and needles. If we had a day without sun downing, I had to go to bed when he wanted to turn in. Sometimes I could watch TV, sometimes not. Joe had become aware that he couldn't follow a plot in a movie or sports. I don't remember having a joyful day of normalcy at any point during the past five years—maybe more than five.

Now, I am home alone, missing the Joe before Alzheimer's invaded him, and also missing my Joe with Alzheimer's. Where and how do I find that simple life I enjoyed so long ago? I hope through prayer somehow I will stumble on that kind of day again. I will never quit looking and praying for peace.

Entry #19

How would I get through the week without family and friends like Carolyne and Ed? They called to see if I wanted to go eat. I wanted to be with someone. We had dinner.

Entry #20

Every day, I get up alone to a quiet house. I sit here, lonely, with no one. Unless there is a miracle cure for Alzheimer's, this is how it will always be.

Joe has long, uneventful days too. The difference is I pray Joe forgets his sorrow. But my sorrow follows me around like a lost puppy. I feel like a balloon with no air. Contentment and joy are rare commodities for me to feel.

Entry #21

I had an appointment with Mary Ann, my counselor. After an hour of talking and crying, I think I will be okay for another week.

Afterwards, I went and visited with Joe. I desire to see him day and night. When I sit close to him, it is almost like nothing has changed. Then, it is time to leave. I always leave with a heavy heart.

Entry #22

Mindy, Joe, and I got a pedicure. We met Stacy, Eric, Jackson, and Haley at the Elite. Joe was confused with that many people. In the future, just Mindy and I will eat with Joe and not expose him to a big group of people. That was more than Joe could deal with at that time. Alzheimer's not only segregates the one suffering, but it affects us all. I was really sad when I arrived back home tonight. I cried hard just like I did when Joe left in May. I wonder if grief is a permanent part of my life.

Entry #23

When I arrived at Sodalis today, Joe began sun downing. When he begins to sun down, I might as well leave. I knew that Joe wouldn't respond to me or any kind of conversation. The problem with me leaving is that I don't want to leave Joe.

Some visits run very smooth when it is time for me to leave; other times the visits don't run smoothly. I usually go around 2p.m. and have a glass of tea while he eats a snack. Then we sit in the den and watch TV until dinnertime. When Joe told me to quit talking loud, I knew it was time to go. There are many times as soon as he sees me, he begins to ask about his car. Joe thinks he has two Oldsmobiles. He has never owned an Oldsmobile. He asks if I have a car, where I parked the car, and then tells me that he is ready to leave when I am. These are always difficult departures. I can't take care of Joe. I want to be with him, and he wants to be with me, but I know it is out of the question.

Entry #24

On one visit, I thought Joe knew who I was when I walked in to have dinner with him. After we finished eating, Joe went to the bathroom. When he came back, he slowed down, put his face close to mine, and asked, "Are you Deane?" He had forgotten I had been with him before dinner. I should have left before he knew who I was, but I wasn't ready to leave him. I am never ready to leave him.

After dinner, Joe and I were sitting on the porch. George, who is a resident, kept walking past us. On one of George's rounds, Joe said, "How are you doing?" George's answer was, "The same as you." Joe got a big laugh from George's reply.

Entry #25

Jody brought Mel, our granddaughter, down to see Joe and me. Mel was hurt when Joe didn't remember her. We ate at Cotton Patch, then bought a Blizzard. Jody and Mel dropped me off at Sodalis, and I stayed with Joe until 9:30p.m. when Mindy picked me up. After explaining to Joe over and over who Mel was, he finally said he remembered her. I like to think maybe he remembers his granddaughter—at least for a short period.

Entry #26

The girls at Sodalis tell me Joe helps in the kitchen, wipes off the table, and helps fold clothes. Joe always helped clean up the kitchen at home, but the last time he folded anything was way back when we folded cloth diapers. The girls at Sodalis told me one night that he sang Kansas City to the group. He received an astounding ovation.

Entry #27

I bought Joe a recliner for the den and a full size bed for his room. I don't think he noticed the bigger bed, but knowing he has a new bed makes me feel better. I was attempting to make his new home as comfortable as I could. I kept thinking, *Joe has worked all his life. He has a king size bed at home, and he deserves better and larger than a twin bed.*

Entry #28

Mindy and I picked up Joe for a haircut. We ate at Casa and stopped for a blizzard on the way back to Sodalis. Joe loves going places. He stops and talks to strangers. He is so happy to be out. Walking out the door alone at Sodalis and getting into the car takes all the energy and fortitude I can muster.

Entry #29

My balance is not good, which is a hazard when living alone.

On Saturday, I climbed out of bed to let the dogs out. To keep myself from falling, I grabbed the blinds. It was like grabbing a razor. I cut my left hand in two places. I finally was able to stop the bleeding and wrap up my hand.

Later, I visited Joe, but I didn't stay long. He fell sound asleep in his chair. I left about 4:30p.m., returning to an empty house.

Entry #30

Our children and grandchildren help make my world go round.

Jackson and Eric picked me up today. We picked up my other four grandsons, and the seven of us went out to dinner. We stopped for a Blizzard before taking the boys home. If Joe had still been living at home, it would have been impossible for me to leave him and go out with our grandsons. If we took Joe, the noise and talking would upset him. This is my tradeoff.

Entry #31

When I arrived at Sodalis today, Joe was showering. When he finished dressing, he joined me to play Bingo. Joe never joins group games or crafts, but today he played Bingo with me. After a few games of Bingo, we sat in the den and watched a ball game. I then ate dinner with him.

By practicing self-discipline, I am beginning to find pleasure doing nothing more than eating with Joe, sitting with him (minus any conversation), and just being.

Entry #32

Today, I was sitting close to Joe in the den at Sodalis. Several of the residents were pacing around the room. Joe was uneasy, continually asking me, "When are we going home?" I stayed longer than usual because the three girls working were very busy. They had several new residents they were getting settled in. One new guy looked in every room, searching for his wife. She came for him around 6p.m. The other two were lost and pacing the floor. Several of the men had to be changed, one cursing anyone who tried to help him. The girls who work there had to bathe two women before bed and give a breathing treatment to another.

As I left around 8p.m., a big full moon was lighting up the parking lot. When it is a full moon, I don't think three workers are enough. A full moon affects the folks. When Joe was Justice Of The Peace and the moon was full, he always said folks seemed to get in more trouble than usual. When the moon was full, it wasn't unusual for Joe to get called to go to the police department to deal with restless criminals.

Entry #33

One Sunday, I brought Joe home to watch football. He loved being here, and I loved having him here. I had to take him to the bathroom many times. Joe and the dogs had a cheerful reunion. After several hours, Joe told me the bookcase looked familiar. Joe walked through the house looking in every room, trying to find something that was familiar to him. I don't think anything was familiar to Joe except for me, the dogs, and the bookcase. As we were getting in the car, he wanted to sweep up the acorns in the driveway just as he did when he lived at home. Joe always made sure the patio and driveway were clean, and he picked up sticks and debris in the yard. Now, unless the yard men are here, things aren't quite as groomed as they once were. But neither am I.

Joe and I took a ride. We bought fish for dinner and took it back to Sodalis to eat. Joe thought we were eating at a restaurant, even though we were at Sodalis. When we finished eating, he was ready to leave and go home. My departure didn't go smoothly. When I told him we were going to watch TV, he told me I was crazy. I knew it was time to leave. After I got home, I called to see how he was doing. Joe wouldn't go to bed—he was waiting for me to come and get him. These episodes are heart-breakers. I tried not to let any of the valleys we experienced erase the quality time we shared today.

Entry #34

On Monday, I picked Joe up to see Dr. Stern. Then Joe had a pedicure and a manicure, and we had dinner at Cotton Patch. We were sitting there, just the two of us, and Joe suggested we get a piece of paper, write down the restaurants we liked, and take turns eating at them. Joe has not had this much incentive in years, and the fact that he was able to relate his ideas was a happy moment. We went back to Sodalis, and Joe was fine when I left to come home to an empty house.

Entry #35

Today, Wednesday October 27th, 2010 is our 59th wedding Anniversary. I had an appointment with my therapist, Mary Ann, and I think my grief is getting under control. Mindy and I took Joe to Casa for our anniversary celebration this evening. On the way home, we bought Blizzards, and were able to leave Sodalis with ease.

Entry #36

Jody came in to town today. He and I had a good long visit before picking up Joe. We had dinner, and visited a while longer at Sodalis. We had an easy departure. When we wear out Joe, he is ready for us to leave so that he can go to bed.

Entry #37

Tonight is Halloween, and I won't turn on my porch light. In the old days, Joe loved answering the door, greeting the kids, and handing out candy. He was never ready to turn off the porch light.

On another note, I tried to zip my jeans today, and had no luck. I must be using food as my comfort. I need to work on that.

Entry #38

I've dreaded the months of November and December. The days and nights are difficult being alone, and it's even harder when facing Joe's 82nd birthday on November 27th, Thanksgiving, and Christmas, which are all family celebrations. I plan to take Joe out for his birthday, and take a cake over to Sodalis. The Waco families will participate. If I brought Joe to our dinner on Thanksgiving Day, it would be much too difficult for him to sit lost in the noise and confusion of people talking and kids running around. Should I go to lunch with our children, or should I be with Joe?

Entry #39

Today, when I started to leave, I told Joe that I would be back later, and he said to me, "I guess I drew the short stick." That statement and others like it make it harder to leave, and cause me to think maybe I moved him away too soon.

I know I am depressed, but I don't want to take antidepressant pills. I am sad. Every day I visit Joe, a part of him that was present yesterday is gone. I think crying is a natural part of losing the man I love. I am not losing him all at once, only one brain cell at a time.

Last night as I lay in bed, I began praying. Out of the blue, my prayers were asking God to forgive me for not taking care of Joe at home. I cried for hours.

Entry #40

Joe has had a few nights of sun downing. Last night, he tried to escape out the front door. I kept calling to check on him, even though I know I can't do anything. I just wanted to know when he finally settled down for the night.

Entry #41

I have to face December without Joe. Should I put up a tree? I don't think I will put up a tree—it will be too hard for me. I would probably drop and break the ornaments with tears blurring my vision. Maybe I will put up outside lights. At least that would be festive without facing so many memories.

Entry #42

Jody brought me two small lighted trees to put on a table. He said that I should have a Christmas tree. I am grateful for my little trees.

Entry #43

I visited Joe often this month. He may be sleeping when I arrive, but when he wakes up and sees me, his face lights up. He tells me how important I am to him and how much he loves me. If only that could take place with us living together at home. Joe usually knows me, but sometimes he calls me Iva. It took me several years not to react to Joe calling me Iva. As soon as I tell him my name after he calls me Iva, Joe says, "I know that."

Entry #44

Whenever I spend time with Joe like yesterday, it affects me the next day. I don't reveal my distress while I'm there, but when I get home, I am emotionally tired from my feet to my brain.

Entry #45

Joe sometimes asks questions like:
- What place is this?
- Do we have a room?
- How much does it cost?
- Do you sleep here?
- Where do we eat?
- Can we drive our car?

I answer his questions calmly, lovingly, but not exactly truthfully. If I said I didn't sleep here and told him how much it really cost to live here, it would upset Joe.

Entry #46

Sunday, I slept late. I guess I was depressed.

The day after I visit, I think of Joe all day. I miss him, but know this is the way our lives will be until one of us dies or I have to move out of our house. Notice that I didn't say "home." This is a house, not a home. I, at 80 years old, barely get around, living here with our two dogs and memories of Joe. I must face the fact that this is my life.

Entry #47

We managed to get through Christmas. Sodalis put a tree up, and Joe really enjoyed the Christmas festivities. He never asked if I had a Christmas tree.

Entry #48

Another New Year's Eve. The first time Joe asked to kiss me was in 1950, and every New Year's Eve will always be a night of memories. I will remember that night and try not to dwell on the present.

2011

Entry #49

We are beginning a new year, 2011. January is a time of renewal, but what do I have to renew?

The day before me is filled with things to do, such as correcting my book, *I'll Be Seeing You*, writing Jody a belated birthday letter, and opening and answering e-mails. But it won't fill the emptiness that I feel every day. I have to face the reality that Joe will never live with me again.

When I met Joe, I was searching for love. Through the years, he has filled up all the sad, empty holes from my childhood. Somehow, I have to find a way to fill up my lonely spots again.

As much as I have to do, I feel misplaced. Even though I have many projects—and these are projects I am interested in doing—I sit at my computer desk and work, yet all the while there is a void in my life. My life is empty without Joe.

While making plans for this new year, to use the pronoun "I" and not "we" is depressing.

Entry #50

Dena and I had a long visit with Joe today, but when she and I started to leave, Joe didn't understand. Joe has always cautioned me about driving in the rain, being careful on highways, and letting me know he just wants me to stay home and be safe. I told him I would call him when I arrived safely back home, and I did. Arlene answered the phone, and she told me that when they got Joe in bed, he told Sue, "Tell my wife I love her." How many times can my heart be broken? I was sad and upset because this is not the way a couple should have to live in the "winter" of their years. Joe should be able to tell me he loves me with me beside him, and I should be able to tell him how much I love him. Should I spend the night with Joe, even though he wouldn't remember the next day? Do I want to spend the night with Joe? In a way, the answer is yes. Being able to touch him through the night and waking up beside him would be wonderful. If I spent the night with him at Sodalis, what kind of questions would Joe ask when we woke up? Would he be upset, wondering who the stranger was in his bed?

Entry #51

This disease keeps me living in limbo.

Entry #52

This time last year, my heart was split into pieces when I moved Joe to Sodalis to live away from me. I wanted to live my days with Joe, but I also wanted a life. As a caregiver, my life was dedicated to Joe day and night. When Joe was at home with me, I didn't have a life.

Entry #53

I cry when I pray, and I cry when I don't pray. I cry just thinking of Joe or saying his name.

Entry #54

Funny the way our minds jump around. I was sitting and thinking about Joe, and suddenly my thoughts were:

Joe is still alive. He may not be the person he was ten years ago, sometimes he may not know me or his own children, but I can still visit him, and I do love him. I can bring him home for a visit.

Every time we are together, Joe tells me how much he loves me. He introduces me as his wife and sometimes as his sister. He loves me, and my love for Joe goes way beyond love.

Joe was more than my husband, lover, and friend. He had become my soul.

Entry #55

Every night, I sit and watch TV. Joe and I may live another ten years, and this is all I have to look forward to—living apart. I had lived a fairy tale love affair for sixty years. I was in love with Joe at first sight, and I knew Joe loved me. Was that enough to sustain me until the end of our lives?

My visits with Joe, his affection for me, knowing I can see him every day, and letting the memories of our time together fill up the hole in my heart will have to be enough during this trying time. I am thankful for the years and love we have exchanged. No one can dim these memories and visions. I am forever thankful.

Entry #56

I've been busy tying up all the loose ends for my knee surgery in March. I've been looking forward to it. What a sad statement . . . my life is so empty and lonely that I'm looking forward to surgery.

Entry #57

The night crew at Sodalis told me that Joe has been getting up lately looking for me. How sad is that? We were both looking for the other one before going to bed.

Entry #58

The other night I was visiting Joe, and he looked right at me, and asked, "Where is Deane?"
I told him, "I'm right here beside you."
"Oh yeah, I forgot."
We both laughed.
I laughed to keep from crying.

Entry #59

The week before my knee surgery, I spent almost every day with Joe. I knew I would be out of commission for a couple of weeks. Mindy was my stand-by in place of Joe.

Entry #60

March 23, 2012 was the day of my double knee replacement, and my cousin Dicque who was like a sister to me died that same day. I am double-grieving—for Joe and for Dicque.

Entry #61

At my surgery, I wasn't scared. I just missed having Joe by my side. Mindy and our boys were by my side when the nurses took me to surgery. Mindy spent two nights with me. I was in the hospital for a week, then another week of rehab. The rehab was very, very painful. Mindy and Jim went to San Francisco, but I was well cared for by our sons. The boys visited several times a day the week I was in rehab. Jody brought me home and immediately went to the grocery store and left instructions for me to follow. I hired someone to stay with me at night for about six nights. Laura was here during the day. I was on a walker until May.

I spent May and June going to rehab. I have graduated from my walker to a cane, and have been driving myself to Sodalis.

Entry #62

Sometimes, I can whistle, and Joe knows it is me. Other times, he acts like he knows me, and I think he does know me, and then 30 minutes later he will look at me and say, "Where have you been? I'm not ever going to let you leave."

When I pay attention and am making notes on a daily basis over the course of a few months, I can see Joe's slow decline.

Entry #63

May 14th was the one-year anniversary of Joe moving to Sodalis. It seems like years since he was home with me. I'm not sure I was thinking long term a year ago when I made the decision to move him. As a matter of fact, I knew I wasn't. Had I faced that this living arrangement was forever until the end, my kids would have had to commit me. While living apart, each day seems more like a week. I know I can't take care of both of us. I pray for Joe to be able to take care of his personal hygiene, read the paper, remember his address, phone number, and have no sun downing. Then and only then, I could bring him home. There's no fault in dreaming.

Entry #64

Most of my visits with Joe are loving and wonderful until it is time for me to leave. But who can blame him? He knows me at times, and somewhere deep in his mind he knows we belong together and he wants to go with me wherever I am going.

One day out of the blue Joe cried, but I didn't know why. Did he want to go with me? Did he even know why he was crying? I didn't handle Joe's tears well. When anyone cries, it brings tears to my eyes. But to see my loving husband cry and not know why or how to comfort him, gave me good reason to cry like a baby.

Entry #65

On one of my visits with Joe this month, he was in rare form. He was singing scat, then he hummed "Taps." He sang most of the time I was there.

Entry #66

I am crying more. It doesn't help to talk to anyone. Nothing in our lives change. Joe and I are not together and never will be.

Entry #67

Mindy and Jim are going to Colorado from middle of June until middle of July. My grandsons Jackson and Eric keep me company several nights a week. Jody brought Blake, our grandson, for a visit. I can't begin to tell you what these visits mean to me. Their visits reinforce the fact that I'm not alone in the wilderness of Alzheimer's.

Entry #68

Joe had a UTI, and that may have been the cause of his confusion and sleepiness.

Entry #69

Today, Joe and I laid on his bed and listened to music. He has an amazing ear. During one tune, he said, "The band changed meters in eight bars."

Entry #70

Yesterday after dinner, we sat in the den. As hot as it was, Joe went outside. Jerry—another resident—sat with him. As I was leaving, they were deep in conversation. To us, nothing they said to each other made sense. But to them, they were in a conversation. Praise the Lord!

Entry #:

In the beginning of Alzheimer's, the jealousy-demon instigated by Alzheimer's often infected my mind, and I would be jealous of Joe's deceased sister. But that doesn't bother me anymore. Through prayer, learning, and accepting more about this disease, I am able to overlook many things. I know Joe loves me, but I have to put this in perspective and remember that Joe has Alzheimer's. I am confident that I am always first in his mind and always have been.

Entry #71

Today, when I walked into the living room, Joe recognized me and was glad to see me. He told me I was his love.

Entry #72

The girls informed me that Joe played Scrabble recently. I was so happy to know he joined with the other residents to play a game. They said he was a good speller and that he was very bright. But we already knew that.

Entry #73

The temperature on this August day is 108-degrees. I had the oil changed on the Lincoln and the tires checked. This is all new for me. Joe always took care of the cars, finances, and big decisions. Being in charge isn't all it's cracked up to be. One should be careful what they wish for.

Entry #74

Barry came for an overnight visit. Joe enjoys Barry and always has. When Barry is around, there is a lot of laughter. Those two laughed and joked for the entire visit.

Entry #75

I visited Joe today—probably because I needed to see him more than he needed to see me. When he told me he was tired of "being like this," it broke my heart once again. Then in the blink of an eye, Joe looked at me and said, "I never thought I could love someone as much as I love you."

I never knew love could be this deep, overwhelming, and painful.

Entry #76

I brought Joe home for the afternoon. He played with the dogs, took a nap, and then we had dinner. I made his favorite—roast and the trimmings. After he ate, he said, "I have never had a bad meal at this table." When I took him back to Sodalis, he asked me if we would ever sleep together again. Then, with a somber look on his face, he asked me, "Are you trying to get rid of me?" If he only knew how much our separation hurts me day and night. I am slowly accepting that our lives will continue on this path of separation. I wasn't thinking forever when I moved Joe last year. I have to face the fact that this will be our normal everyday life until the end of our lives. In order for us to live a full life under these living conditions, my job is to find a way to accept and learn what is best for both Joe and me. That is a tall order!

Entry #77

For my 81st birthday tonight, I had dinner with Joe at Sodalis. I repeatedly told him that it was my birthday, and each time I told him, he gave me a birthday kiss. After Sodalis, I went to Dena's for dinner to celebrate.

Entry #78

Tonight, I ate dinner at Sodalis with Joe. After dinner, we were sitting in the den when a fight broke out on the porch. All the workers ran out to break it up. A new resident was sun downing. Joe was in the bathroom, and I knocked on the door to see if he needed anything. The new guy was walking toward me, and I put up my hand to stop him. That only made him more mad, and he approached me faster. I locked Joe and myself in the bathroom, and waited for the new guy to walk away from the bathroom door. But he stood close to the door. When I didn't come out, the new guy hit another resident in the head and scratched a worker. I decided to bring Joe home with me for the night.

When we got home, we watched TV, had cookies and a drink, and went to bed. I was feeling a joy I hadn't felt since Joe moved a year ago. He remembered the side of the bed he slept on and informed me he couldn't sleep on the other side. I had him roll over to his spot, and we settled in for the night. Joe hugged me several times, kissed me goodnight with each hug, and we fell asleep. I lay in bed thinking, *I can bring Joe home! I can do this! I am able to take care of both of us!*

The next morning was a different story. Joe couldn't find his toothbrush sitting right in front of him, he couldn't find the toothpaste, and he couldn't put his legs in his pants or comprehend that his shoes were in front of him. I had to squat down (after knee surgery) and put his pants on him. Then, while we read the paper together at breakfast, Joe thought the dogs needed to be corrected, but they weren't doing anything.

I realized that, as much as I love Joe and as much as I enjoy him being at home with me, I couldn't take care of him at home. Being a caregiver to Alzheimer's in this stage is a 24-hour job. Our children might disown me if I took on that role again. This is the pits in which I will live until one of us dies.

Joe didn't want to go back to Sodalis, but he went with a happy face. When we arrived, the girls came out to meet him, and he was fine and was happy once he got out of the car. I went in with Joe, and we had an enjoyable afternoon.

I stayed at Sodalis to make sure the new guy had some help with his sun downing. I discovered that the doctor had prescribed medication to the man, even though the wife didn't want him medicated. Hopefully in time, the new resident will be acclimated to his new surroundings.

Entry #79

This month, I went to Dr. Grayson for my yearly female exam. When I left Sodalis, I told Joe I had to go see the doctor for my annual Pap test. He told me, "Good. I'm glad you are taking care of yourself." He understood Pap test. Alzheimer's constantly amazes me.

Entry #80

Every day is a short funeral when I have to leave Joe behind. My life will never be the same. I must find something to fill up my days besides sleeping.

Entry #81

Every day, I wish Joe was standing at the door to the study here in our house, waiting for me to finish writing like he did before I moved him. But that will never happen again. How do I go on knowing Joe is alive and just across town? I am alive, but we have to live apart?

Sometimes I fantasize about how our daily lives would be without Alzheimer's. I would not be alone day and night. I am sure our days would be much the same as mine are now, but I wouldn't be alone. Joe and I would go to sleep together and wake up together. When I was sick, I was afraid of being alone. If only it had been possible for us to live out our lives together and if one of us was ill, we would watch over the other. That would be Heaven.

Entry #82

I received a call from Sodalis yesterday saying that they found Joe flat of his back on the porch, and he said that he had had a heart attack. I called Dena to come and get me. We met the ambulance at Hillcrest and after five hours in the ER, we took Joe back to Sodalis. Getting Joe in and out of the car was extremely difficult and is a whole other story. I should have known that Joe didn't have a heart attack, because this wasn't the first time he had fallen and said he had had a heart attack. Joe told the girls he hadn't fallen down, but that it was a heart attack. Joe was confused and funny at the same time. In the car taking Joe back to Sodalis, he talked nonstop. He asked if he was dying. He asked Dena and me how he would know it if he died. We didn't know whether to laugh or to cry. Joe was confused not understanding why he went to the hospital or what was happening to him.

On the way back to Sodalis, he used the f-word. Dena said, "Daddy, I have never heard you say that word." He told Dena, "I won't say it again." Even in the grip of Alzheimer's, Joe still desires to honor his family. At times like this, we overlook the years of respect and example Joe gave to his children. If every woman could say to their Daddy that they had never heard that word from him, it is a tribute to his children and a great tribute to the man. Joe was a genteel person and a gentleman in every way. He still is.

Entry #83

It is going to be difficult to get through our 60th wedding anniversary on October 27th. And then, of course, the entire holiday season that follows.

Entry #84

A virus recently went through all the residents and workers at Sodalis, except for Joe. Or so we thought.

When Jody and I arrived at Sodalis to take Joe to dinner a few weeks ago, Joe was in his chair in his room and not alert at all. There was no communication between Joe, Jody, and me. Joe got up to lie down on the bed, and his diarrhea was like water with no control. We called for an ambulance to take Joe to the hospital. We spent the next six hours in the ER. Joe was X-rayed for pneumonia, and the test showed that he had pneumonia. The urine sample was so bloody, it was impossible to get any results. I hired someone to stay with Joe overnight.

When we arrived at the hospital the next morning, the sitter gave us an update about his night. This continued for over a week. Joe was unable to understand all the tests that the doctors were running. My heart ached for him. I wished I could help him understand. I wished I could somehow give him comfort and security. The doctors wanted to run many tests that were invasive.

Our thoughts were: *We are not going to put Joe through a lot of tests. If it was conclusive that he had bladder cancer, we would not agree to chemo. Joe has Alzheimer's. His life isn't going to improve whatever the results. The fact is that Joe is going to lose more of his memory as time goes by, and Joe will be less likely to understand why he is having more tests. Alzheimer's is a death sentence. Modern medicine can't fix it.*

As a family, we decided we would not put him through these exploratory test.

After running a urine test, the result was a kidney infection. The proper antibiotics were ordered, and, after staying in the hospital over a week, Joe was released. An ambulance took him back to Sodalis. I wasn't sure Joe would recover. But as usual, he was up walking around within a few days. Witnessing this man's determination and his spirit to beat the odds is remarkable. As I watch Joe wrestle with this disease, I am not ready to give him up.

Entry #85

I am so thankful Thanksgiving and Christmas are over. I find every day difficult having to live without Joe by my side. These three months have been about keeping my head above water. I could drown in despair if I didn't look for some joy in each moment. You may have to kick over a rock to find joy, but it's around us if we look for it.

2012

Entry #86

Last night, I heard myself praying. I heard my voice, and I shocked myself. Was that my voice? And why did I thank God for Joe's memory loss?

When it is time for bed, I go through my nightly rituals. I put our dogs, Abby and Alison, out for their last potty break, close off their room, give them their nightly treat, turn off the heat, put on the security alarm, take care of my personal nightly duties, and get in bed. As I was tucking myself in last night, I said, "Joe, here we are—you at Sodalis, and me alone in our bed." Then I heard myself thank God that Joe has no memory of living here. I paused and asked myself, *Was that my voice?* It was.

Never in my life would I have thought to thank God for Joe's loss of memory. I immediately knew why I had said that prayer. If Joe's short term memory was intact, he would be sad every day like I am. Since he only has memories of long ago, then he forgets new things almost immediately, making it easier for him and for me. Alzheimer's is a wicked, stressful disease but how comforting it is to the family that their loved one has no memory of what happened today or yesterday and no knowledge of his brain being destroyed by the plaque and tangles that are demolishing his brain. There is always something for which to be thankful, even when suffering with Alzheimer's.

Entry #87

Jody, Blake, and J. J. came for a visit. Joe didn't know who our grandsons were, but he knew he was connected somehow.

Entry #88

Every night, I find myself sitting here at home alone, wondering what purpose I have in life without Joe. I have no responsibility, except for me and our dogs. I've often tried to think of something to do besides watch TV. What should I do to get free from this mindset?

All day every day at home, I am stuck in limbo between life and death.

Entry #89

I get up out of my chair in the den with tears rolling down my face, and I go to sleep alone on my side of our king-size bed. I have nothing to look forward to tomorrow, and nothing that I did today had any meaning except my visit with Joe. I wonder how I can live my life without Joe, but I know that I must find joy for Joe's sake and also for my sake so that I can be emotionally healthy for Joe. He is in the world of Alzheimer's without me, and I am alone here in the real world. He couldn't be in my world again, and I don't know how to enter his world. We are stuck in separate worlds. My marriage vows give me strength to be by Joe's side no matter what obstacle is put in our way.

Entry #90

I am so thankful Joe doesn't miss me like I miss him. Every minute of every day, there is a great void in my life. I know this will not improve, so I try to cherish the days Joe knows me as soon as I walk in. As soon as I walked in yesterday, he told me I was pretty and that he would tell the world. Joe knew I was someone close to him, but I'm not sure he knew I was his wife. He had no recollection of our life together.

Entry #91

Joe was in a good mood today when I visited him. I was straightening up his closet, and when I stepped out from behind the closet door, he looked at me with a big smile, and asked, "Where have you been?" I knew it would be hard to leave, so I stayed for dinner. Joe asked his usual questions: "When are we leaving?" and "Where are we going?"

I had taken suckers to Joe, and I asked one of the girls to get him one before I attempted to leave. When he was zeroed in on the sucker, I was able to leave without him noticing. He seemed content with his sucker. I don't remember the last time I was content. Contentment sounds foreign to me.

Entry #92

One day when I visited Joe, I whistled as soon as I walked in. By the time I arrived in the den, he was up looking for me. The Joe before Alzheimer's was waiting for me with a big smile on his face. I find great joy in his smile, in his kisses, and in his open arms.

Entry #93

Every Friday, a group of college students from Baylor visits to play bingo or paint with the residents. This past Friday, Joe painted and was deep into his project. He painted only different colored strokes. One part looked like he had written fish or dish. I put it on the front of my refrigerator. Is this sad? Hell yes, but I find joy sitting with him while he paints.

Entry #94

Today, I was telling one of the workers at Sodalis about trying to talk to an investment firm and how the firm couldn't find my last fax. Joe was nearby and picked up on what I was saying. For almost two hours, he wanted to make a call. He didn't know to whom, and he didn't know the phone numbers, but he was stressed trying to take care of this piece of business for me.

When Joe is lucid, trying to live in the world outside of Alzheimer's is stressful for him. I can't help him understand, and at the same time, I don't know how to relieve his mind.

Entry #95

This afternoon, I took Joe for a ride in the car, and we listened to music. I had to keep reminding him that it was him singing and playing the trumpet on the CD. At one point, he said, "That guy singing stays in tune, and he's really good." He listened to his own trumpet solo, and after one tune he said, "That is as good as it gets," never realizing that it was him playing the trumpet. I will cherish the memories of today forever. I just wish that both of us would cherish this day and not just me alone.

Entry #96

Joe met me in the hall today. He knew I was special without being able to verbalize "wife" or "Deane," and he told me that I was a pretty woman. I told him that I had to be pretty to snag a handsome, sexy guy like him. Is he more lucid lately than normal? I have to remember that Alzheimer's, the wicked disease that it is, gives the caregivers a false sense of hope.

Entry #97

Again, Joe wants to go home. But home to him is where he lived when he was a ten-year-old boy. Home to me is where Joe and I lived together. I told Joe that I can't take care of him, and his answer to that was, "I can take care of myself."

Entry #98

The sun was shining today, and it wasn't too cold. Joe and I sat outside, and he enjoyed his Blizzard. He knew me, but not as his wife. Joe's libido is off the charts for an 83-year-old man. I have read somewhere that men with Alzheimer's think of sex a lot, and he does. If

I'm honest, the one thing I miss most is the intimacy and sex we both enjoyed. That will never happen again, but the memories of our love will have to be enough.

Entry #99

Barry came to visit today. He and Joe were outside walking, enjoying this late April weather, and Barry asked Joe when he got so old? Joe's answer was, "Isn't this awful?"

It's good to find humor in these things.

Entry #100

June has been a stressful and sad month so far. Francesca and I took Joe to see Dr. Stern. Francesca told the doctor about Joe's daily sun downing and how he's been loud and vulgar. Dr. Stern prescribed Depakote. Over the next few weeks, Joe's dose was increased to the point that he slept most of the time and couldn't walk or feed himself. In the middle of June, he went to the Emergency Room with a UTI. He was in a bad state, sleeping and non-responsive most of the time, but still showing a sense of humor when he did respond. Mindy and I agreed to put Joe on hospice because of his condition.

Joe didn't eat or drink anything for four or five days. His only water was on a sponge to wet his mouth. I sat in Joe's room, watching him. I would crawl in bed with him, telling him, "You're not alone. I'm here with you." After two rounds of antibiotics for a UTI, and decreasing his meds down from five a day to one in the morning then to zero, Joe began to return almost to where he was before the UTI.

I was sitting with Joe reading a book (really, more like staring at the pages). During the previous five days of the ordeal, I had shifted my mindset to the fact that this may be the end. But out of the blue, Joe rallied. I asked if he was thirsty, and he said yes. I asked him if he was hungry, and he said yes. I asked him if he wanted to eat in his bedroom or go to the table. His answer was, "I want to go to the table."

Joe was back.

In less than three weeks, Joe was shuffling along, feeding himself, and singing.

Entry #101

Stacy, our granddaughter, was climbing Mount Rainer and had a bad accident. She fell fifty feet and had to spend the night on the mountain with two rescue rangers. The helicopter had been able to rescue the other four climbers, but the weather prohibited Stacy from being rescued. The next day, the weather was bad, and she had to walk down, which took her seven hours. She was safe, nothing broken, lots of cuts and bruises, but in fairly good shape. Her mom, our daughter Mindy, will carry this fear with her for a long time. Stacy, hopefully, will reflect on this close call before climbing again. This was just something else to worry about besides Joe and Alzheimer's.

The word stress doesn't come close to labeling my anxiety. Stacy was in danger, Joe was on hospice and not very responsive, so to comfort myself I fed my stress with candy, cookies, and ice cream. By the end of June, Stacy was going back to work, Joe was slowly getting better every day, and I had ten pounds around my middle to remind me of how I used food for comfort all month.

Entry #102

During the past 10 days, Joe has been sleeping a lot. He isn't interested in drinking or eating. We all try to get him to drink water so he won't get another UTI. Should I stay with him at night?

Entry #103

The Daveys from our church came to Sodalis to offer Communion to Joe and me. I introduced them to Joe again. He sat quietly for a minute, and said, "Seems like I've met them somewhere".

Entry #104

When I go to Sodalis, I never know which Joe will be present. Today, Joe was the Joe of September 1952 when he met me at Orly Field in Paris, France for our second honeymoon. Oh, yes Alzheimer's was present, but it never darkened our visit. I always knew that Joe was in love with me. Today, he verified that his love for me is the same as it was 60 years ago. I was presented with the hope diamond of joy.

Entry #105

I took a cake to Sodalis tonight to celebrate Joe's birthday. I took him a shirt and encouraged him to open his present, but instead of opening the gift, he said, "I don't think so." The cake and ice cream was uppermost on his mind—*not* another new shirt. In the past, Joe would have been more interested in clothes than cake.

Entry #106

A quote I read today: "Count your joys, not your foes. Count your blessings, not your woes."

Entry #107

Alzheimer's is a horrific disease robbing the person of memories and talents. Today, Joe was lucid and crying and said, "What have I done?" I froze, but I knew he was looking to me for comfort. He didn't know how to finish that statement, but I knew what he meant, *"What have I done in my life to cause me to have this kind of life?"* Joe looked at me, and said, "The only thing I know to do is jump off a building, and he quickly told me, "Don't worry I'm not going to jump." I didn't know how to answer or comfort him. In the tiniest part of my brain, I thought, *Why don't we both jump off a building together and put an end to this life living in the land of Alzheimer's?*

Entry #108

Sodalis had a Christmas party for all the families. Joe was annoyed by the noise and all the people. He ate in silence, looking around the room, not knowing where he was, who all these people were, and not even knowing who I was. Joe feels close to me, but that is about all.

Entry #109

The day after Christmas, I think Joe may have known me. I received many kisses and hugs during my visit. I was grateful we finished 2012 with only a few very stressful days. Most of my days, I am stressed simply because of knowing that for the rest of my life Joe and I will live apart.

Entry #110

Around 11p.m. last night, I called Sodalis to check on Joe. Reagan said he was walking and talking. He wasn't sun downing bad, but most of the night he roamed the halls. I remember those nights when Joe lived at home—no sleep, just waiting for Joe to leave that zone and come back to bed.

I wonder if he suffers anxiety during these spells. I hope not. I pray that during these times God is helping Joe across the river to a better place.

Entry #111

I visited Joe today, and he was sleeping. I gave him a hug, told him who I was, gave him a kiss, and he never opened his eyes. I sat there for maybe thirty minutes, then I told him I was leaving and would come back when he woke up. With eyes still closed, he said, "No, I don't ever want you to leave me." I sat another thirty minutes or more, then left. He never asked where I went or had any memory of me being there. Sure, my heart was heavy when I left, and it took me a couple of hours sitting in my chair at home to recover from my emotions, but I brought home my gift, and that was Joe saying in his sleep, "Don't ever leave me." I will never leave him. We had talked many times about our hearts being one, and he told me he always felt close to me even if he couldn't say my name. My life's gift is Joe. Will life go on? Yes. And the gifts that are always present in my life will give me reason to live a full life for Joe and my family.

2013

Entry #112

As we begin 2013, I wonder what this year has in store for us. Will Joe continue to decline? Will the decline be slow or fast-paced? Will God take him home? Will a cure for Alzheimer's be in our future? And will I continue to be strong enough to get through another year?

Entry #113

I have given myself permission to miss several days in a row of visiting Joe.

One day recently, he was humming, and I told him the title of the song he was humming. I said, "I love this tune—'Body and Soul.'" He was happy to finally know the name of the tune. Even though he remembered the tune, he had forgotten the lyrics and title of the song. Here was a musician that had played for 70 years without music or lyrics, and within five years had lost his memory of the one profession he loved. Joe laughed and continued to hum, and his happiness at knowing the title of the tune was obvious. I couldn't wrap my brain around this fact. Joe Johnson, playing and singing since the age of fifteen without music or lyrics, and he didn't know what he was humming. This would make any of us think about jumping off a building.

One of his regular golfing buddies, John, recently told me a story: He and Joe were playing golf, and John asked Joe, "If you had to give up either golf or your trumpet, which would you give up?" Without any hesitation, Joe said golf. Joe loved golf, but I knew from our earliest time together that music was his first passion. I am thankful I am his passion too.

Entry #114

I called to see if Joe was awake, but he was sleeping. At about 5p.m., I called again. Eva said Joe was up, but that he was sun downing and would not come to the table to eat. I told Eva I would see him another day. I sat down to watch TV, but I got the feeling I should go see Joe. Something kept nudging me. So I took him some chips, a banana, and a Snickers bar. When I arrived, he was on the porch kicking little pieces of debris off the porch with his foot. If he didn't recognize me as his wife, he did acknowledge me as someone he knew. We sat on the porch in the rocking chairs, and Joe ate some chips, the banana, and the Snickers. He was sun downing a little, but he was not anxious. After an hour, he wanted to go inside. We sat on the couch together. He wanted my purse, and I knew that meant he wanted more candy. Watching this disease destroy a life tears one's heart completely apart.

Entry #115

On a recent visit, Joe began to tell me a story about being drunk. He said that his being drunk was going to be put up on the screen for all to see. He told me he was sorry, and he knew it was wrong to get drunk.

I told him, "I have known you for 62 years, and maybe ten times have you drunk a little too much. You haven't done anything wrong."

He said, "Yes, I have done something wrong. And you were drunk too."

I started to defend the both of us. He was sun downing, and I knew the best thing was to go along with the story. And so that's what I did.

In spite of the story about being drunk, we had a great visit. He sang and kissed me over and over. When I got home, I realized that today, May 14th, marks three years since Joe and I have lived apart. I'm facing another night alone in the king size bed. Maybe I'll invite my two dogs in for company.

Entry #116

Stacy, our granddaughter who fell on Mount Reiner last year, has fallen again. Mindy and Jim, her parents, just left for Scotland. Mindy received the call right before she boarded the plane. Stacy's twin brothers flew to Colorado to stay with her in the hospital. Mindy came back to Texas, and Stacy and the boys flew back. I have no idea why Stacy keeps climbing—what is so addicting about climbing rocks? Stacy will be recuperating for six weeks. This is just another stress for me.

Entry #117

It's now August, and I visited Stacy and Mindy for the first time since they've been home. It was a rewarding visit in many ways. Our imagination does dirty tricks on us, usually imagining the worst. Stacy was propped up, talking and smiling, and she seemed accepting of the long recovery ahead of her. I sat with her chatting, then minutes later I noticed a picture Mindy had taken of Joe with Holly, our schnauzer. The minute I saw that picture, uncontrollable tears came flooding.

I have seen Joe just like that with the same expression holding our children and the thousands of times I cuddled up with his hand on my head just like he was holding Holly. This same look is on Joe's face at times when I visit him when he gives me a kiss or lays his head on my shoulder. Joe looks at me with compassion that fills up all the empty spaces. Living with this disease, you grab on to anything no matter how small or insecure to fill up the pain of reality. It was me and Joe in that picture. I couldn't control my tears.

I had Jackson turn the picture toward the wall. Eric came over to sit with me. It is one of the most powerful pictures of Joe I've ever seen. In that picture, his love and tenderness is prevalent.

After I went to bed, I had to make myself not think about the picture. Even now, days later, I am moved to tears when thinking about the picture. It is a moving picture of this loving man, but I don't want a copy. I have that image seared into my mind, for I have seen the same expression for almost 62 years. The picture is worth a million words.

Entry #118

I didn't take my own advice today when I visited Joe on my birthday. I took a cake to Sodalis, and I imagined a visit where Joe, the residents, the personnel, and I would sing "Happy Birthday" to me, have cake, and then I would cuddle with Joe. Joe did sing "Happy Birthday" jazz style, but that was it. He talked about another woman and wanted to take me somewhere safe. When Joe lived at home, it wasn't unusual for him to tell me there was a woman there that claimed to be his wife, and that he didn't want me in our bed. Joe was afraid the other woman would cause a problem finding me in his bed. I wonder if that was what he was thinking today.

All afternoon, he kept patting my arm and telling me to go. My expectations were off the wall, and my disappointment brought me to tears. That was when Joe wanted to take me to safety and told me I needed to go. I left crying, both sad and angry with myself.

I questioned what part of me would expect Joe to be himself. He has Alzheimer's, and I made matters worse by fantasizing about my own birthday with Joe. I guess all caregivers have a lapse of judgment—either that, or we don't want to face reality all the time.

After an afternoon of tears, my girls and grandchildren had a party for me at the Elite. Facebook was popping with greetings from family, friends, and Facebook friends I don't even know. There is joy every day, but I just have to look beyond the Alzheimer's to experience it.

Entry #119

I have noticed a change in Joe the last few days. He is lost in thought with his eyes closed and not at all present with me. I often feel like the man I am sitting with isn't Joe. He looks the same, but he's different. Still, I love this new man just as much as the old Joe. My memories will have to be sufficient enough to last until the final curtain closes.

Entry #120

I had a wonderful visit with Joe today. I sat by him, put my arms around him, and he said to me, "This is a good day." I told him every day with him is a good day. We need a cure for Alzheimer's—if not for Joe, then for our children (since Alzheimer's is genetic) and for the multitudes of others who may be susceptible.

Entry #121

Our 62nd wedding anniversary on October 27, 2013 came and went. Always being a romantic, I wanted Joe back for at least that one day, but ol' Al is forever present.

Entry #122

I wrote the following for our local newspaper this month . . .

What is Alzheimer's?

Fifteen years ago, when the public heard a news story about Alzheimer's or saw an article in print about Alzheimer's, they more than likely just glossed over the story. Today, it is different.

Since my husband was diagnosed 10 years ago, I have had to face the fact that death is imminent, yet slow. There are no shots, medications, or surgeries that give us hope. There is nothing. We are doomed to watch our loved one's memories dissolve before our eyes. Life goes on, and the family must find a way to endure this wicked disease.

I try to live in the moment. I look for joy in a wink, kiss, or simply holding his hand. I know this: Joe may have Alzheimer's, but that is not who he is. Joe is my husband of 61 years. He is father, Boppa, musician, Justice Of The Peace, Lawyer, District Judge, and a man of honor and humor. This is the man I love.

I know there is no cure, but I have faith that our communities and country will help find a cure with the necessary funding. I plead with our government to help the millions who are suffering now and the millions who will hear the diagnosis in the future.

I am honored to be this year's Spokesperson for the Alzheimer's walk in our community. My family and I live with this disease every day, hoping for a cure. It is too late for Joe, but the necessary research could help countless others in the future.

-Deane Johnson

Entry #123

Jenna, the Hospice nurse, called earlier asking permission to draw blood from Joe. Hospice had asked for an update saying his last reports were good and that maybe he didn't need to be on Hospice. The first call was around 10a.m. Jenna called back an hour later to tell me that Joe was a sick boy. He had fever, a bad respiratory cough, his urine was bloody, and she couldn't draw blood. The blood coagulated as soon as it was in the tube. She called Dr. Stern, and I called my daughter, Mindy. She picked me up, and we went straight to Sodalis.

Every time Joe gets sick, I shift my thinking to, *This could be the end.*

Joe was sleeping when we arrived. He wanted to get up, but he couldn't stand by himself. Mindy and I made him stay in the bed. Joe was hungry and ate some Jell-O, soup, and ice cream. Soon after, he was sleeping soundly again, and I knew David who worked nights would call me if need be, so I decided to leave. Mindy took me home at the end of this long, stressful day. My world of Alzheimer's is changing daily. How do I meet the changes and find joy?

Entry #124

The way Joe bounces back to his old self is always a surprise. If only the plaque in his brain would respond to his good immune system in the same way. Because of my tremor, I can't help with feeding Joe, and my balance isn't good, so I am fearful of us both falling if I try to walk with him. I am really no help to the staff, but I want Joe to know that I am with him and will stay close to him for his comfort and security and mine too.

Entry #125

Today, I went to see Joe, and he looked great. He kissed my hand, and said, "I love this woman." Then he kissed my hand up to my elbow and back again. He did this four or more times. I took that joy home with me afterwards, but I also took my sadness as well. With tears streaming down my face, I drove home.

The only person in the world that I want to discuss my surgery and battery-problems with is Joe. My children are interested and caring, and my daughter Mindy is always by my side. For this, I am thankful. My husband, Joe, would be by my side too if the albatross of Alzheimer's wasn't around his neck.

I do have a choice, and that is to kick the sadness to the curb and only bring the joy home with me. The tears and sadness could be my constant companions, but I refuse to let myself drown in sadness. God has given me the ability to journal every day, publish a book, make decisions, and live a full life with memories of 62 years as Joe's wife.

Prayers and love keep me going . . .

Entry #126

Joe turns 85 today. Sodalis gave him a cake, and the residents gathered around the table for cake and punch. Our daughter Mindy, her husband Jim, our other daughter Dena, and three of her four boys came. We sang "Happy Birthday" and took lots of pictures.

Looking for the right words, Joe complimented his grandsons and patted his daughters telling them how pretty they were. The girls and their families left. Joe was whistling "Happy Birthday" the entire night until he fell asleep. I enjoyed seeing his response to the family.

My usual comments as I went to bed were, "You, at Sodalis. Me, here. And nothing will change until one of us goes to live with God."

I shook myself and said, "If all you are going to say is negative comments, no wonder you are unhappy."

So I began to list all the things I am grateful for.

Entry #127

On Sunday, December 1, 2013, I convinced Joe to sit with me on the couch. He asked me if he could hold me. "Yes and forever," was my answer. I laid my head on his chest, and he wrapped his arms around me and softly said, "Now I'm at home."

Tears flooded my eyes. I shed tears of joy for the love we share and tears of sadness for what we lose every day.

It takes talent to be a caregiver to Alzheimer's. You have to learn a new bag of tricks every day. I know that I am Joe's security and his comfort, just as he is still mine in many ways. I am able to take home the love we share and not allow sadness to destroy the joy. Who ever thought one could shed both tears of joy and sadness at the same time?

Entry #128

Today, I told Joe that I can't walk because my knees hurt. He immediately said, "I thought you had that fixed." I had to laugh, knowing that somewhere in that brain of plaque and tangles are memories. Joe somehow remembered that I had knee surgery almost two years ago.

Entry #129

I don't call to talk to Joe, fearing that my voice may cause him sadness or to wonder where I am. Yesterday, the phone rang, and when I answered, Joe's voice replied. I was greatly surprised. He was crying, and my mind was searching for some way to quiet his tears.

I told him, "I love you," and he repeated "I love you" back to me. He was still crying, but my voice helped him some. Maggie got on the phone and told me that Joe was sitting around the table singing, "I'll See You in My Dreams," and suddenly began to cry. She asked him if he wanted to call me, and he did.

Entry #130

Christmas was just another day for Joe and me. We had the usual dinner of turkey and all the trimmings, but it was just another day.

I did not do a good job of following my own advice, which is:

Don't visit with expectations.

I anticipated a long and loving visit, and I left disappointed.

I did get to sit with Joe for a while on the couch, with him resting his head on my shoulder. Even though my expectations were not met, just holding Joe and hearing him give out sighs of comfort, was the joy I will always remember. I've told myself so many times, *If you wait quietly and let yourself be in the moment, you will find joy.*

2014

Entry #131

It was a full moon tonight, and half of the residents at Sodalis were sun downing.

Joe was in the shower when I got there. Anyone who has Alzheimer's hates to shower. They have no memory of showering, and every time Joe showers, it is like his first exposure to a shower. You and I know the sequence of showering, but the Alzheimer's person doesn't. The water is either too hot or too cold, and their skin may be sensitive to temperature changes. They have to be guided through lathering up, shampooing, rinsing, and drying off. Then the next thing is for someone to put a towel on them. The staff wants to get them dried off and dressed quickly. At this point, the patient is upset and usually quite vocal.

Joe was mad when he came out of the bathroom tonight. He looked at me, and nothing registered with him. I had candy, and when he finally sat down, he began eating his candy while sitting on the edge of the couch. After a few minutes, he leaned back, ate the other piece of candy, and was quiet. I don't think he ever knew who I was. He just knew I had candy and was able to sit for a long period of time. He was relaxed, very quiet, and attentive to eating his treats. I sat with Joe for five hours until dinner time. Eventually, he stood to go have dinner, and I left to go home.

I left knowing that Joe had felt secure by my being with him, even though he never said anything to me but just put his hand out for another treat. I hope he also felt the love I have for him.

Entry #132

One day this month, I revisited Joe's and my early courting days. Joe, in his special way, took us on a trip back in time.

When I arrived at Sodalis, the first words out of his mouth were, "I hoped you would come." We were in the living room with other residents and visitors. Joe met me, and I got a lover's kiss, not the usual sister kiss. Wow! We sat, walked around, and sat down again. Joe's inhibitions had disappeared. He was tender, and he told me, "I love you all over," and we spent the next couple of hours loving each other, using words of endearment and insinuations. During the visit, I wondered if I should cover us with a quilt. Joe was courting me. Nothing happened, but Joe remembered all the right places to touch.

Entry #133

Shortly after I moved Joe to live apart from me, he told me that when he went to bed, he talked to me. Living with sadness, disappointment, anxiety, frustration, anger, loneliness, and emptiness I realized that loving deeply helps erase all of those feelings, but I must kick the crap to the curb so I can wrap myself in the love we still share and always will.

Entry #134

Our grandson, J.J. Johnson (Joe Johnson III), stopped by on his way back to Houston today. I told Joe who he was and that J.J.'s daddy, Jody (Joe Johnson Jr.), was our son. From the way Joe connected, I knew he felt an attachment to J.J. Joe patted his back, then looked into his eyes. I could tell that Joe knew him in his own way.

There is heartbreak in every visit. I have to find a way to experience joy in each visit.

Entry #135

Every visit is different to a degree. The day Joe told me that he wanted to see me more often caused me to question if I visit him enough. Does he think this thought often? I want to always be there for Joe when he needs me.

Entry #136

God spoke to me through Joe . . .

On March 25th, my visit to Joe was about the same as all other visits. Joe was napping. I sat close and hugged him. He told me he loved me. I brought him a Snickers and a Peanut Planter bar. He was eating his Snickers, and said to me, "You're always thinking of daddy." That sentence said a lot to me. I began thinking, *As a young wife, I always kept score and would have expected him to be thinking of me if I was thinking of him.*

My mind was spinning. From Joe's comment, I received a lifetime gift. He was saying that he could depend on me as I had depended on him for years. I heard from this statement how special I am to him, the comfort and security we enjoy from each other, and the love he had for me. This was a pure gift, no bows or wrapping paper. It is a memory to last a lifetime.

My mind didn't stop there. I began to dissect relationships, thinking about the pronouns we use when talking to our mate. I realized that we always use "me" and "I," but "us" is overlooked. The God-light came on. "Us" and "you" should be the only pronouns we use in making a decision with our mate or anyone. When using the pronoun "me," one will never find a solution that is best for the marriage. I believe "me" and "I" should be eliminated from our relationship-vocabulary, including friendships. Only use "you" and "us." Using "us" is the only way to assure your mate you want the best for both of you.

Entry #137

Yesterday, on Wednesday the 26th of March, I made a speech at Baylor about my book, *I'll Be Seeing You*. I told about my seven years of being a caregiver to Joe while he's had Alzheimer's.

During the hour, as I spoke, my eyes went over the class, but one young girl stood out. I told the class what Joe said when he was eating his Snickers, telling me "You always take care of daddy." The pronouns "you" and "us" had nothing to do with my book, but I needed to share this with the class, and I did at the end of my talk about Alzheimer's.

There were lots of tears—not just my tears, but many students. Afterwards, all the students came to me, thanking me for speaking to the class. Several members had grandparents with Alzheimer's. It was an awesome hour. The pretty young girl with the blond hair was the last to give me hugs. She had big tears streaming from those pretty eyes. She told me she was newly married, they were having some trouble, and until she heard me today she didn't know what to do. She told me listening to my story she knew what she should do to help her with her husband and her marriage. I hope it does.

Entry #138

Joe has a lot of congestion. On my way to see him today, a black cat ran across the street. I wondered if it meant bad luck. Joe was sleeping in a room that wasn't his. He had been up most of last night. The nurses told me he didn't like to go to his room. That is where they change him, and they wondered if that was the reason. I don't think so. If I mention his room, he doesn't know where it is, even though he had slept in this room for years, and I have to show him where it is when I'm there. Just like I have to tell him that he eats in the dining room. I think staying up most of the night happens in the later stages of Alzheimer's.

I sat by his bed for over an hour just looking at him. I talked to God. I thanked God for pairing us up, grateful that I have been his wife taking care of him with Alzheimer's. Thanking God for the many years we've been together (63 years in October). I told God that Joe was a good, faithful man. God knew that. Joe has always treated all people equally, was always ready to explain to his clients about an autopsy, or court ruling, and he would listen to their questions and comments for as long as they had questions. I thanked God for Joe's musical talent. Of course, God knew everything I was saying. I sat admiring this man I married. I reminisced about our life together, talked about our children, his friends, and our grandchildren who will have to get to know their Boppa through stories we tell them. I asked God to take him soon back to the man with no anxieties, no plaque or tangles, who had no memory of this disease, never felt lost, and had his memories back. Heaven will be his Glory. Death is a Gift.

I told Joe that after he departed this earth, I would grieve and miss him, but I would celebrate our life together and all his and our accomplishments. I told Joe that when he reached the Pearly Gates, Peter would hand him a trumpet. Waiting for him would be Nick Klaras on drums, Rusty McNeil, Bobby Hamilton, Tommy Norwood, Jack McDaniels on sax, Ed Burleson, Butterball Ferguson, Dick Smith on bass, and his Casa Blanca guitarist. These guys will get to jam with Stan Kenton, Glen Miller, and Woody Herman in Heaven.

Entry #139

When I arrived at Sodalis today, Joe was coming inside from taking a nap on the porch. I wondered if he knew who I was. I like to think he did, because he kissed me and said, "I love you, darling." Maybe at that moment, he did know me or at least sensed a closeness to me.

Later into the visit, I told him, "I'm your wife." That seemed to upset him. In the early days of sun downing if I told him that, his answer was "I don't think so."

We sat down on a couch together. I knew there would be no conversation with words, because Joe began losing his nouns a couple of years ago. Instead, he patted me. But when I tried to hold his hand, he would kiss my hand, put it back in my lap, and cross his hands. I reached for his hand a few more times and got the same response.

There I was, sitting with the love of my life, sorting through all these feeling, but having to accept that Joe had no feeling for me or memory of me in that moment. Thus, my joy for the day was his kiss when he first saw me and said, "I love you, darling."

There are seven stages of Alzheimer's, and I am often asked if I know what stage Joe is currently in. I have no idea how to figure that out. Most of the time, he is in the "zone," then in the bat of an eye he is lucid and seems to know who I am.

Really, what difference does it make? No matter what stage of Alzheimer's our loved one is in, we caregivers adapt and love with all our heart through all the stages.

Entry #140

Joe can only shuffle along now. It's not his normal walk. He still feeds himself, but his vocabulary is for the most part gone and he doesn't like to bathe or shave. I stopped being able to have conversation with him about a year ago, but every once in a while he has a lucid moment and is the Joe before Alzheimer's.

Entry #141

At this time, I am wondering why Joe is still taking Exelon and Namenda daily. I don't want to give him a drug that would prolong this world in which he exists. Maybe to some, that sounds harsh. For eleven years, I have lost a piece of Joe every day. Every time I leave, it is like leaving his funeral. I live knowing today is the best Joe is ever going to be. From today on, he will spiral toward his inevitable destiny. I ask myself if this is the way I would want to live out my final days, not knowing my family, not knowing where I am, not knowing how to read or write, not able to follow a TV show, and completely lost in the vast, empty world of Alzheimer's.

Entry #142

If Joe is thirsty, he doesn't know how to ask for a drink. He may be in pain or hurting somewhere, but he can't tell us where. If he wants to do a simple thing like blow his nose, he doesn't know how to ask for a Kleenex. That is not the way I would want to live, and I know my Joe—smart, talented, a man filled with pride, and a man who lived life with excellence every day—would not want that either. My question is, *Why keep giving him meds to slow down the memory loss of Alzheimer's? His memory for the most part is gone.*

Joe physically looks the same, but he is a shell of the man he once was mentally. I don't know what to do for him. Should I ask our doctors to stop the meds? I need help. This is a lonely world in which I live.

Entry #143

Many people wonder why I visit Joe so often. My visits are as much for me as for Joe.

Entry #144

When I arrived at Sodalis today, Joe was sitting on the couch with another female resident. The aides asked her to move to another chair so that I could sit down, and she adamantly refused. Joe stood, and this lady stood and put herself between Joe and me. He had an infected toe, and I didn't want her to step on it. Her habit was to come close to

Joe and kiss him.

Unbecoming to me, a streak of jealousy raised its ugly head inside of me. Knowing better, but not thinking clearly, I told her, "No."

Finally, the workers led Joe to a couch, and positioned themselves between Joe and the resident so that she wouldn't step on his toe.

This lady circled us, trying to get close enough to pat Joe. All the while, I was trying to protect his foot. When she stopped in front of Joe, I asked her to back up. On one of her rounds as she passed us, she said, "You have him now, but he is mine."

Thankfully, the jealousy I once harbored disappeared. I reminded myself that this woman is sick with Alzheimer's like Joe. There are three other male residents, and she is just as attentive to them as she is to Joe.

I told myself it is time to look at the humor in this situation and stop being a mother lion.

Entry #145

Joe's right toe has hurt him for almost a year. At first, I thought it was gout, then an ingrown toe nail, but time has proven us wrong. Last week, Joe was diagnosed with gangrene. There isn't anything that can be done at this time. Amputation or a stint for circulation is out of the question. If either were done, it wouldn't improve his quality of life. Joe doesn't have diabetes, no circulator problem, and he doesn't smoke. The podiatrist said he was sure it was caused by a blood clot.

Entry #146

We are entering another stage of our lives. I think from today onward, it is an era of wait-and-see.

Entry #147

I was at Sodalis on Sunday, as I am most days. I sat by Joe marveling at his good looks and sweet demeanor. He was sleeping, and I was telling him all the things we would be doing if the plaque and tangles had not invaded his brain. We would go to church and sit in our pew. Probably drop by for a burger or chicken on the way home. We'd have our usual Sunday night dining out with friends. Joe would play golf, sweep the patio, take his evening walk, we would go to Super Slow to exercise, watch TV, and in the evening have our nightly cup of coffee, floss our teeth, then go to bed next to each other. These are some of the thousands of memories I will cherish and long for.

Entry #148

As I have in the past, I will lean on God, our family, and our friends as we wander down this unknown path. I feel I must be strong for our children and grandchildren. They have known Joe as "Daddy" and "Boppa," and now they try to find Daddy and Boppa, and he isn't there anymore.

Entry #149

I will treasure this day Joe gave me a lover's kiss, not a sister kiss. I find it difficult knowing we will never have intimacy again. I accept this finality of married life and will treasure all kisses, pats, or maybe nothing more than just sitting and watching him sleep.

Entry #150

It's now early June 2014. When I arrived home today at 5p.m., I felt numb. We finally got Joe on hospice after mass confusion. Mindy took care of everything. When she walked in the door at Sodalis with drinks for all and a comforting smile on her face, I knew that she would take care of everything, and she did. I knew I couldn't make decisions as well as she does. I realize I am not as assertive as I should be. Maybe it was knowing that Mindy standing tall by my side allowed me to shrink from responsibility. I want our children to know I would never shrink from my duty, but today it was too much for me. Tomorrow is another day.

Entry #151

Today, Joe whispered to me "We will be together forever." I know this love that began when we said our vows never ends. It gets more powerful year after year.

I know in my heart that this may be the last time Joe feels close enough to me to respond as my husband. I marvel that the love that has grown during these last few years of Alzheimer's has given me a chance to love Joe at the highest level I could love someone. This is a different love than a husband's and wife's love. It is much deeper than that. I accept and am grateful for this journey as a lesson in love. I don't require anything from Joe to assure me of his love. I am content and warm inside just being with Joe, sitting quietly and nothing more. I don't have to be kissed or hugged to know that this kind of love is deeper than a kiss and a hug. I thank God for showing me the love I've found.

Entry #152

As I approached Joe to give him a kiss today, his eyes were blank. He didn't know me. I have always known this day would come.

Entry #153

Joe couldn't call my name, yet he told me in his babbling vocabulary he loved me and repeatedly kissed my hand. I sat with him for a couple of hours watching other family members who were visiting come and go. Most left with tears in their eyes. As I greeted each one, I felt a kindred love for them all. All of us were on this same heartbreaking journey when we first met. We were strangers in the beginning when we moved our loved one to Sodalis, but now we all are as connected as a family.

The only thing I do for Joe now is bring him candy, keep ice cream cones on hand, and love him. As a wife, that doesn't seem enough. I wish we could share the intimacy we once shared. These memories, prayers, candy, ice cream, and loving visits are my only contributions to the man I love.

Entry #154

All my visits with Joe are much the same, but also different at the same time.

Today, I was sitting right next to him, and he wanted to know where his wife was. Several years ago, this would have made me depressed, but today I viewed it positively. He didn't know I was sitting next to him, but he knew he had a wife. Dee, a staff worker, told me that one evening Joe was walking around the facility, shouting, "Deane, where are you? I love you, Deane!"

Joe may not recognize me, but he hasn't forgotten that he is married to me.

Entry #155

Joe's first love is music, but recently I've noticed that he doesn't listen to music being played on the stereo anymore. Either he doesn't hear it, or his attention is elsewhere.

On Friday, my grandsons, Eric and Jackson Wren, brought over an iPod and earphones, and they downloaded music I had picked out. Then the boys and I took the music device over to Sodalis. Joe was sleeping, and at first there was no response. He listened, made some sounds, and that was about it.

The next day, with iPod and earphones in hand, I made another visit. Joe and I sat on the sofa for over two hours listening to music. For those of you who aren't married to a musician, their way of responding to the music is different than the average person. In the early years, I was surprised when musicians laughed when someone was playing or improvising, but in time I figured out that their laughter was their way of applauding what the musician was playing.

I spent two hours with Joe watching him and listening to him. I thought he would respond more to Sinatra with Count Basie, but his favorites were the North Texas Lab bands, the North Texas Jazz Singers, and Take Six. Joe and I have been going to Denton since 1970 to hear the bands and Jazz Singers. I don't know much about music or harmony. The harmony of Take Six, Jazz Singers, Four Freshmen, Hi-Los, and The Singers Unlimited is different than other harmony. You won't find a jazz musician that doesn't like it.

I cherished sitting with Joe and watching him enjoy the past and the present through music. Joe hears every note, and follows all the improvisations. How can I tell? Because he hasn't changed at all in 70 years of listening to music. Thank you, God, for Joe's talent and for him being able to enjoy the talent you gave him.

Entry #156

The first thing people usually ask me is, "Does Joe still know you?" Most of the time, I think he does.

Recently, one of the girls at Sodalis asked Joe if he was married, and he didn't know. He was told that his wife's name was "Deane Johnson," but that didn't register. Anna said, "Ask him if his wife's name is Loduska Deane Johnson." Joe smiled, repeated my name, and added, "She is a hot babe." I think he knows me from way back when. That is good enough for me.

Entry #157

For 11 years, I have watched this plaque destroy my husband's brain. His decline has been slow, but now is speeding up. Joe's vocabulary used to be vast. Now it is all but gone. He may say four words that I can understand. He had a great walk, now he shuffles. He was a great joke-teller, now he doesn't know what a joke is. He knew how to make me feel special, now his only words are "Thank you, darling" after I have given him a piece of candy. Those words make me feel special. If in some way I comfort Joe, I too am also comforted. It's amazing that we finally appreciate the smallest things, and I believe it is because we are learning to live in the presence of Alzheimer's.

I am now Joe's candy lady. You may ask how I continue to visit when Joe doesn't know me as his wife. My visits are as much for me as for Joe. I don't require any more than just sitting with him, no matter what mood he is in. I receive pleasure when I give him pleasure and security whether it is giving him candy or just sitting with him. When I have made the moment better for Joe, it is a perfect moment in time for me. For now, that has to be enough. I cannot go into his world, and he hasn't been in my world for seven years. Love has to be enough at this stage, and it is enough even though it is emotionally painful missing the man that was. I continue repeating this truth: *Joe has Alzheimer's, but that is not who he is.*

Entry #158

My birthday was on August 17th, an 84-year old female still trying to go full speed. I got up on that cloudy Sunday morning, missing my Joe, had my coffee, and my next stop was my computer. I knew I would have something to read, even if it was an advertisement. Not only did I have 50-plus birthday wishes, but received messages yesterday and today. There is a saying that, as you get older, if you can count your friends on one hand you are blessed. We can disregard that saying. To my friends off Facebook, my friends on Facebook, my friends in Texas, my friends in other states who know me from my book, and my friends in England who wished me a Happy Birthday, I send hugs to all of you. Even though I miss Joe every day, because of each one of you, I am never alone. Thank you all.

My day began with a call from my granddaughter, Stacy, then calls from my sons and other grandchildren. My daughters and their families took me to dinner. Mindy made the traditional great chocolate sheet cake, and I declared my birthday complete.

Entry #159

Today, Joe walked the halls, screaming, "Dena!"
I went to him, but he told me "no" in a loud, harsh voice.
The girls finally convinced him to go into the living room, and I put on a Sinatra CD which calmed him. He dozed, and in his twilight of dozing, he repeated these words to me "I love you to pieces."
Every time I leave Joe, I question myself if I left too soon.

Entry #160

I found myself in a dark place up against a dark, steep, rugged mountain a couple days ago. I couldn't find a way to go over or around the dark mountain. I began feeling defeated, depressed, desperate, and hopeless. The darkness in the room was suffocating.

I lay there in bed trying to figure out how to escape those dark feelings. Was there any way to help Joe escape this dungeon he finds himself in? My mind in that dark place was working overtime. I wondered if I could put Joe in the car and drive us off the double bridges into the lake. We would both be free of this darkness, disease, and hopelessness. A few nights ago, I wondered if I could put rat poison in a Snickers bar. I hope all of you know I wouldn't do either, but this is how our minds work when we find ourselves in this dark place, and my lover is in the deep struggles of Alzheimer's.

Sunday, I was still in that dark place. I screamed and cried most of the day. My wailing turned to sobs, and I asked myself if I was losing faith. My tears rolled down my cheeks like a flood when I questioned myself about my faith.

I am not going to lose my faith yet. I need to give these despondent feelings to God. It is time for me to give my pain to God, seek joy, write my "gratitudes," and be patient with life.

Entry #161

The next morning, after my dark meltdown, I came to my computer, and my message board was overflowing with "thinking of you" messages. I received phone calls from friends of 60 years ago and a lady that worked for me when our children were toddlers called out of the blue. God nudged a friend of my children who surprised me with dinner. Also, a fellow I dated 63 years ago called. He and I doubled-dated, back in 1951, with his parents going to Casa. He reminded me on the phone that he wanted to dance, and I wanted to see Joe. I assured him that I wanted to dance too. He was a great dancer. A friend sent flowers saying, *Just thinking of you*. Our minister came by, as did a new minister I had just met. This was not a coincidence. It was God tapping each one of them to come to my rescue. God's presence is constant, but many times I didn't sit still long enough to feel the presence of God. I was trying to spend time every day sitting quietly, meditating, and listening.

Entry #162

This October day is the "walk day" for Alzheimer's. It is raining nonstop, but nothing will stop our family from walking for a cure for Alzheimer's. Since I am on a walker, I borrowed a wheel chair. Mindy, Jackson, Eric, Dena and her boys, and Jody drove down from Dallas to join in the walk. My kids situated me in the wheel chair and tried to cover me up as best they could against the rain and cold. Off we went and walked the whole way. This was a tribute to my one-of-a-kind husband and their dad.

I wonder if Science will ever have a clue as to why the plaque and tangles begin forming and clogging the brain. If research figures that out, then maybe a cure will be on the horizon. I don't have any confidence that the research will find a cure in my lifetime.

Entry #163

This is a letter I wrote at the end of this year to our Representatives in Washington, asking for them to vote for more funds to end Alzheimer's:

Dear Representatives,

    I am Deane Johnson from Waco, Texas.

    I want to encourage each of you to remember the fight of the millions suffering with the wicked disease of Alzheimer's and vote for more money for research that will help wipe out this disease.

    My husband, Retired District Judge Joe Johnson, was diagnosed only months after he retired in 2003. Unless you have been on this journey with a loved one, you have no way of knowing all that we face with this disease 24/7. You may think that the one who finds themselves in the grip of Alzheimer's only forgets phone numbers, appointments, and family members' names. That doesn't begin to cover what this tragic disease does to the individual. In stage 6 and 7, families must face the reality that everything your loved one has accomplished in their life is gone. My husband has lost his vocabulary to speak. He has lost the ability to ask for a drink when he's thirsty, a blanket if he's cold, or a tissue if he needs to blow his nose. They are waiting to die with no hope. To be honest, I will look at death as a gift. That will be the day our loved one will be freed from this torture chamber.

    I invite you to see what life is like while blindly dealing with Alzheimer's. My book, I'll Be Seeing You, is a day-to-day journal of Alzheimer's with Joe and me. I had to self-publish, but with no advertising families here and in Europe are buying the book. I hope you will purchase it at Amazon.com

    I know our country is in need of many things. Instead of funding less urgent research such as how the Salamander mates, I beg you to fund Alzheimer's. You are our last hope for curing this disease. It won't help my Joe, but it may help the millions of Baby Boomers who will surely face this disease in the coming years.

                                  Lovingly With Tears And Anguish,
                                              Deane Johnson

Entry #164

Every Thanksgiving and Christmas, I am faced with the same dilemma: Do I eat with Joe, or do I eat with my family? I have eaten with him on these special days since I moved him to Sodalis.

On the day we unwrapped gifts, Joe wasn't interested. I kept reminding myself that he is in the latter stages of Alzheimer's. Earlier this month, Santa Claus visited. When Santa sat by Joe, Joe started crying. I am glad I wasn't there to see his fear.

Alzheimer's sucks.

2015

Entry #165

What will we face with Joe in this new year? I was happy when December 31, 2014 came to a close. The holidays from October 27th until the New Year were depressing.

At times, I cry hard, and scream in the privacy of my four-wall house. How long can a person grieve and still retain their sanity? My grief began in November 2003 when Joe was first diagnosed. I have lost a piece of him every day for eleven years. How much more will I lose before I tell him goodbye for the last time?

Entry #166

When I leave at dinnertime, Joe is content with a kiss goodbye, or sometimes I leave without telling him. Leaving without saying goodbye is not as much a problem anymore as it was in his early days at Sodalis.

Entry #167

Sometimes Joe reacts to my voice, but not today.

I told him my full name—Loduska Deane Johnson—and received no response. Then I told him, "I'm your wife." But still, nothing.

I asked if he wanted candy, and he reached for it. But it was obvious he did not feel a closeness to me, and he had no idea I was his wife. For thirty minutes, Joe ate his candies, Coke, and bottle of water with his eyes closed.

Then suddenly, he picked up my hand and kissed it like I was royalty. That was my joy for today. I left crying, trying to figure out a way to find a little happiness in the world of Alzheimer's.

Entry #168

For the past few weeks, whenever Joe sang, it was scat. Today, he sang "Red Sails In The Sunset." I have never heard him sing this song. I think this was a memory from his childhood when he was somewhere around eight or ten years old. Mary Holiday, who worked for Waco and announced acts at the Kiddie Matinée on Saturdays, took Joe weekly to ladies' clubs to sing for them back in 1936. I knew he sang "Tumble Weed," but not "Red Sails In The Sunset." I enjoyed imagining him as a little boy.

Entry #169

Today, Joe wanted to sit in my lap. I surmised that he was in a mental state of maybe two years old. The first time he got in my lap, the aide eased him back onto the couch. Joe immediately got up and sat back in my lap. I motioned for them to leave him in my lap. Joe managed to put his head on my shoulder and sank into the vast empty space of Alzheimer's.

When I knew he had fallen into a deep sleep, we eased him back onto the couch. He kept his eyes closed the whole time. I don't think he ever knew I was there, but I got to hold him on my lap a short time. I believe that Joe regressed to a toddler stage when he wanted in my lap. I was brought to tears knowing that with Joe in my lap, I experienced his time as a toddler on his mother's lap. Now, he was on my lap. When I left, he was curled up on the couch sleeping. I left with tears rolling down my cheeks.

Entry #170

I never miss a moment of memorizing Joe's body language and all of his expressions. In the end, these pictures in my mind and my memories will be all I have left.

Entry #171

Joe has been more affectionate than usual these last few days. When I was sitting beside him, he told the workers attending him, "I love this girl." I put his head on my shoulder, and he dozed off. After his nap, he got up and forgot me again.

His words "I love this girl" fill my heart with security and comfort. My love for him grows deeper each day. For my sanity, I have had to hold on to the few loving words, pats, and kisses throughout these past eleven years of Alzheimer.

Entry # 172

For 11 years, I have watched this plaque destroy my husband's brain, facing the reality that death is imminent. His decline has been slow, but now it is speeding up.

Entry #173

When Joe is lucid for half an hour, I return to the false hope that he isn't in an Alzheimer's stage all the time and I can take him home to live happily ever after. Then, in the bat of an eye, Joe looks at me with that lost look in his eyes and brings me back to reality.

Entry #174

When I went to visit Joe on January 30th, I anticipated it would be very much like my visits in weeks past. But before I got in the front door, I heard him screaming. The screams were different than his screams when workers try to get him to stand up for some reason.

Maggie, the Administrator, met me at the door telling me that Joe was in pain. When he woke up that morning, he couldn't stand up. He was in a recliner when I arrived and had been given Hydrocodone, but that was not enough to soothe his pain. When he hollered and was screaming in pain, he reached for his right leg. He had told a girl in the office that he was dying. I asked him if his leg hurt, and he nodded yes. I asked if he hurt in the groin, and he didn't respond.

When Joe was aware that I was sitting with him, he wanted to kiss me, and he said, "I love this girl." He was pale white, in great pain, and none of us knew what to do. I told Ashley, who was sitting next to him, that I wasn't going to call our children until later. She suggested I call and let them be the judge of waiting to hear from me or coming now.

I had already asked Maggie to call Mindy. Mindy's intuition had been working overtime, and she was pulling up in the parking lot as they spoke. She called Dena, and it was then "wait until" time.

Our doctor informed us that a blood clot in the leg moving slowly was extremely painful. From Joe's screams, we knew he was in great pain. Ashley was sitting with Joe, and from the look on her face, my heart stood still. I sat with Joe asking him where he hurt. All he could do was grab his leg. For a short moment, he sensed my presence and leaned up to give me a kiss. Ashley made the comment that even suffering with that awful pain, he knew me. That spells Love to me. In between his outbursts of pain, his last words were, "I love this girl."

At about noon, Joe was given morphine every two hours, and he finally escaped from his world of pain and fell asleep. Mindy and Dena and I were by Joe's side all day until our sons arrived. Jody and Barry came from Dallas and arrived at about 8p.m. I was going to stay, but our children insisted that I go home that night while they took turns sitting with Joe at his bedside.

I returned to Sodalis early on Saturday, January 31st. It was a long day. Our minister, Leslie King, came by to comfort us and say a prayer. We were with Joe all day, waiting. Yes, we waited for Joe to take his last breath. I had been preparing myself for this day almost from the day Joe was diagnosed in 2003. Or so I thought. We all knew this was the end, and as hard as it was to say goodbye, I looked at his death as a gift.

The sun set and the room grew dark with only a small lamp glowing. Later that evening, our children said to me, "Dad's eyes are open." I sat on the bed with him, talking and kissing his face and neck. I knew these would be the last kisses and loving words I would share with him. After a few minutes, his eyes closed. That moment was the last time I held Joe close, telling him he wasn't alone, reassuring him that I was with him.

I stood and sat in a chair very close to his bed. A few short minutes later, our children said, "Dad's eyes are open again." There wasn't a sound in the room. No one was weeping. Joe looked up at the ceiling and slightly behind him. His eyes were wide open and his mouth opened, as if he was going to say something to someone. Suddenly, the biggest smile grew upon his face. It was an ear-to-ear grin that stayed for a moment, then he took his last breath. We witnessed Joe seeing the light of God. This was a magic moment for our family.

At that moment, he was free of the plaque and tangles in his brain that had kept him in an Alzheimer's dungeon for over eleven years. Joe left this life as he had lived it, giving peace and grace to his family with those eyes wide open and the biggest ear-to-ear smile I have ever seen. I was there to witness the gift of death. I sobbed the moment he took that last breath, and my sobs could be heard around the world. Joe was my life, and now there is only half of me left to finish whatever God has for me to learn and do.

> *A good name is better than precious ointment,*
>   *and the day of death better than the day of birth.*
> *It is better to go to the house of mourning than the house of feasting:*
>   *for this is the end for everyone, and the living will lay it to heart.*
> *Sorrow is better than laughter, for by sadness of countenance,*
>   *the heart is made glad.*
> *The heart of the wise is in the house of mourning.*
> *But the heart of fools is in the house of mirth.*
>   *-Ecclesiastes 7*

Entry #175

It has been months since Joe's death, and I am sharing with you my days and months of coping after his departure and after us both finally being free of Alzheimer's.

Joe found peace joining his heavenly family on January 31, 2015. I left Sodalis saying goodnight to a group of people who had become my family for almost five years. I was overjoyed seeing workers called back just to say their goodbyes to this great man of distinction. The hall was crowded with friends and workers at Sodalis. After Joe's last breath, my tears and loud sobs filled the room and overflowed into the hall. The end of Joe's life was a moment when we knew that he had seen the marvels of Heaven and at the exact moment of his last breath, I knew I would be alone until I saw the same light he had seen. A perfect departure would have been if we both had "seen the Light" at the same moment, but I am left to travel the rest of my life solo.

I didn't want to watch the funeral home come for Joe. One of my children took me home, but I don't remember who it was. Dena went home to be with Austin who had had to postpone the celebration of his 18th birthday for another day. Mindy wanted to spend the night with me, but I told her I was fine, and I was. Jody spent the night. I got ready for bed and went to sleep. Isn't that strange? My husband of sixty-three years and three months had died, and I simply came home and did my normal nighttime rituals and went to sleep not shedding a tear.

On Sunday, February 1, 2015, we met at the funeral home to plan the service. I don't know whether I was stoic or numb, but I picked out the casket and made funeral arrangements, and I did it all dry-eyed. I had intended to have Joe's obituary already written and was sure I could knock it out in no time. I sat down at the computer, listed family members, Joe's jobs, music career, Army, marriage, and accomplishments, but it read more like a to-do list than an obituary. My mind was frozen. This would not do. I had to write an obituary, but not in a list form about his life. My daughter Mindy, my son in-law Jim, and my twin grandsons Jackson and Eric wrote the obituary.

 I didn't think I could keep my grief under control at the visitation, but I did, greeting friends with a calm demeanor. This was unlike me. God put his hand on my shoulder and was with me for three hours, giving me strength until the last visitor left.

 Joe's burial was the morning of February 4, 2015 at Oakwood Cemetery. I was more than touched the moment when our oldest grandson, who had not been at the visitation, viewed the casket in tears. The family was gathered around Joe's casket that cold winter morning, listening to our minister, Leslie King, comfort us with God's words. The military flag was presented to me, and I tried to remain calm. But in the back of the room came a soft cry from our six-week old great-granddaughter. It was a symbolic cry that was a message to her great-grandfather, saying, "I don't know you and will never sit in your lap, but I am here and will love you from the stories I will hear about you." I got through the burial feeling the warmth of God and family.

 The next hurdle to jump was the memorial service. Our son, Barry, gave the eulogy, transforming a sad occasion into a celebration of Joe's life. Joe's music played as friends flowed in. The laughter was spontaneous listening to Barry's Joe Johnson stories. Our minister, Leslie King, comforted our family with a perfect tribute. Dr. Stern played a trumpet solo of "How Great Thou Art." Then there was the Lord's Prayer, and the exit music was "Smile When Your Heart Is Breaking." The memorial service was a happy sendoff.

<u>Entry #176</u>

In the weeks and months after Joe's funeral, I found myself standing in a desert, alone for the first time in my life with no compass, no incentive, and no Joe. It was time to put my life back together, and I am still figuring out how to accomplish that. You see, my life is made up of two parts: before Joe died, and now after the funeral and what to do with the shock. I must face the world without Joe and figure out how to live with only our memories.

It has been a year since he departed. For the first three to four months, I couldn't cry. I never felt any burning in my eyes, not one tear. I just went through the days telling friends, "I'm fine," but I knew that this wasn't normal. Friends said that because I had grieved for eleven years, I had grieved enough. I knew that wasn't the reason I couldn't cry, but the reason was unknown to me.

I was sad losing bits and pieces of Joe, but now he had died. Before the final curtain call, I could see him, kiss him, and maybe he would have a minute of lucidity and we would connect as we once had. I had hung on to the "maybe moments" for over eleven years, but now it was over and there were no tears.

Several years ago, Mindy took a picture of Joe holding our dog, Holly. When Joe was at Sodalis, I could not look at the picture without falling apart seeing the compassion on his face.

Recently, I asked Mindy to bring me the picture to replace the one of Joe and me after he was diagnosed with Alzheimer's. I could no longer look at the picture of Joe and me after his diagnosis, because I didn't see the *real* Joe—all I saw was Alzheimer's. The picture of Joe and Holly taken at the beginning of Alzheimer's reveals the compassion Joe exuded all the years I knew him.

To all who will be facing grief in the future, I urge you that when you say your final goodbye, be prepared to face the stages of grief. When death arrives, allow yourself time to grieve. You'll experience shock, and even numbness, in the beginning. Then when your defenses are down, your grief will begin.

Entry #177

As a young wife, I had loved Joe, but I remember my needs through the years to be put on a pedestal. Even after being married for 50 years, I loved him but wanted him to think of me with flowers, cards, and gifts.

As we grew older, we were greatly looking forward to Joe's retirement. But with his diagnosis, I had an awakening, and it was a depressing, startling wake-up call. While living in the land of Alzheimer's, I was introduced to a deeper, unconditional, maternal love. I had to learn to simply be in the moment with Joe, having patience to live in the moments of no connection with him, putting him first and appreciating the smallest gestures of his affection. His last words—"I love this girl"—have been a great gift to me. Money can't buy the lessons I've learned living beside Joe with Alzheimer's.

Life is a celebration. I said goodbye to Joe for eleven years, which were the first five stages of grief. I will grieve for Joe in many ways until I join him. My love for my soul mate grows and is stronger than I ever imagined. After this journey with Alzheimer's, grief is an old friend, but it's different now than it was in the years after Joe was diagnosed.

When Joe and I went to Europe years ago, we recorded tapes each day about our outings. Recently, I listened to the tapes from Italy and Paris. I thought listening to his voice would trigger a tear, but Joe was so funny, I laughed.

Entry #178

I received permission from Bill Tinsley to share his poem. I used the pronoun "he" instead of "she" . . .

Where did he come from,
This man who walked into my life when I was young,
Who joined his life with mine and all the time,
My life was joined to his?

I bore our children, we raised them,
And he taught them by his example, how to love by loving me.
How did this happen, that he became more than my lover and my friend,
That he became my very soul?

Entry #179

This book does have an ending. For almost twelve years, all my documented days included Joe and me. Now, all I have to write about is me and grief, me being homesick for Joe, and me meeting this solo-side of my life positively. Somehow, I'm managing my days and nights aware that my soul mate has left me. The love I have *for* Joe and the love I have *from* Joe is a love affair I never could have imagined in my wildest dream. I am left to survive alone. With God's guidance, I hope to make a difference in everyone's life who faces a journey with Alzheimer's.

I faced all the challenges and found grace.
Deane Johnson

Entry #180

I Now Know What Love Is

I thought I knew what love was
From the moment I first laid eyes on you.
Each time I saw you, my heart skipped a beat,
And when I was with you, I would find myself speechless.

I thought I knew what love was
When I saw you waiting for me at the altar.
My knees were shaking, and my heart throbbing
As I walked toward you.

I thought I knew what love was
When we had our babies one-by-one,
And sharing the indescribable love two people experience
When raising their families.

I thought I knew what love was
As I watched each child grow,
Unique in their own way
Blossoming into young men and women.

I thought I knew what love was
Experiencing the bittersweet love we felt
The day our daughters were married,
And giving up our sons when they took their brides.

I thought I knew what love was
Waiting to welcome each grandchild into our family,
Then each time they crawled on my lap,
Giving me those wonderful, sticky baby hugs.

Recognizing how lucky I am as I watch you sleeping in your chair,
I now know what love is.
It is not the accumulation of things,
But making do with what one has.
It is not houses, cars, vacations, and money.
It is family and friends.
Love is making memories when nothing special is happening.
Love is letting go.
Love is accepting and sharing.
Love does not need to control.
Love is not jealous.

Now I know what love is
When feeling your foot searching for mine
In the middle of the night,
And feeling your hand on my back
To make sure I'm breathing.
Now I know what love is.

Entry #181

I knew you when I was only ten.
I sat in my room alone dreaming of the kind of man I would marry.
I knew I wanted a man who would love me unconditionally,
Even though I didn't know what that meant.
I wanted Love.
I dreamed of a house with a big yard.
I wanted babies and lots of them, as well as animals and family vacations.
I would sit for hours thinking about you.
I knew I would find you someday.
I knew my dreams would come true, and so I dreamed on and on.
When I walked into Casa Blanca, I knew I had found my dream.
And so I had.
There you were singing with the trumpet under your arm.
Our life has been a dream come true, our "Magic Carpet Ride."
I never was ME until I married you.
Children and grandchildren have enriched our lives.

Entry #182

We find ourselves in the winter of our years,
Loving as we did in the beginning.
Sixty-three years living my dream that came true.
Now I'm alone, but I still have a dream and that is:
The day you are standing in the bright light
With arms outstretched waiting for me.
Life is enriched by our dreams.

Joe's Obituary

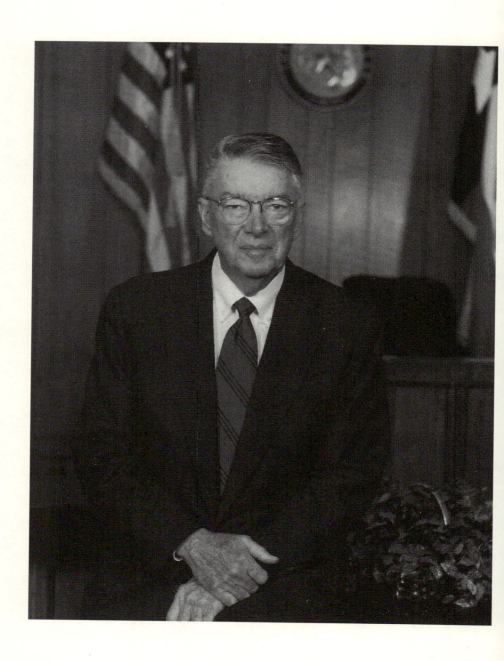

Longtime Judge, Joe N. Johnson, Dies

(credited to Tommy Witherspoon, and published in the *Waco Tribune Herald*)

Joe N. Johnson, longtime McLennan County state district judge and justice of the peace, died Saturday after suffering from Alzheimer's disease for more than a decade.

Johnson, 86, who affectionately called the McLennan County Courthouse "The Rock," went to work in that historic building for 40 years, serving 24 years as justice of the peace and 16 years as judge of 170th State District Court.

He was diagnosed with Alzheimer's the year he retired. But before that, Johnson combined his love for the courthouse with his love for music, playing his trumpet at the 100th anniversary of the courthouse in 2002.

Prior to graduating from Baylor Law School in 1964, Johnson made quite a name for himself traveling the country playing trumpet with the Art Mooney Band, the Sunny Dunham Orchestra and others.

Johnson was about 10 years old when he found his older brother's cornet among a pile of junk the family garage. Soon, he was playing tunes. By 15, he and some children from his Waco neighborhood formed a band, and they eventually became the house band for Mary Holiday's Kiddie Matinee, which was broadcast on WACO radio every Saturday during the 1940's.

The band played clubs around Waco until Johnson was 19, when he got an offer to jump to the big time. The Sunny Dunham Orchestra, which Johnson had heard on the radio, asked Johnson to join them at the Roosevelt Hotel, New Orleans' finest at the time.

Leaving Waco for the first time, Johnson was living in the French Quarter and playing for a top-name band.

After that, the band hit the road with Johnson in tow, playing the ballroom circuit in the Midwayst, Chicago, St. Louis, and New York. The band played at the Roseland Ballroom in New York, the site of Ed Sullivan's Harvest Ball, and Johnson said he could have stayed in the Big Apple to pursue a full-time career in music.

"I had a God-given talent, and I have no doubt I could have gone as far in the music business as I wanted," Johnson once told the Tribune-Herald. "But a man must make an election."

"If I had grown up in Las Vegas or New York, it might have been different."

Instead, Johnson said he chose "home, family, and stability, and caught a train back home to Waco."

The choice was fortunate for the citizens of McLennan County whose lives Johnson touched in 40 years of public service.

"Judge Joe Johnson was always welcoming to the lawyers and litigants who appeared before him in court," said 54th State District Judge Matt Johnson, who is no relation. "When tensions were high, he had the ability to put people at ease with his kind-natured sense of humor and quick wit. His decisions were based on the law, but he always tempered them with ordinary common sense. Judge Johnson served honorably, ethically, and with integrity during his 40 years on the bench."

Judge Ralph Strother, of Waco's 19th State District Court, said Johnson served as a mentor to him.

"Judge Johnson was still on the bench when I assumed office," Strother said. "He was a friend and mentor to me. I took to heart some sage advice he gave me: 'Don't let being a judge go to your head, and don't take yourself too seriously.'"

As Johnson battled Alzheimer's, his wife, Deane, turned her daily journal chronicling the challenges they faced into a book, I'll Be Seeing You: A Wife's Journey With Her Husband's Alzheimer's. *She said she hoped the book would be a help and comfort to others in similar situations.*

She said she planned to donate half the proceeds from its sales to the Alzheimer's Association.

A memorial service for Johnson will be at 11a.m. Wednesday at First Presbyterian Church. Visitation will be from 5 to 7p.m. Tuesday at Wilkirson-Hatch-Bailey Funeral Home.

To view the video of Judge Joe Johnson's memorial service . . .

1) Visit www.WHBfamily.com
2) Scroll down, and search the obituaries for "Joe Johnson"
3) Click on "Judge Joe Norman Johnson, Sr."
4) Click on "Photos & Videos"
5) Click on "Webcast Video" to view a celebration of Joe's life

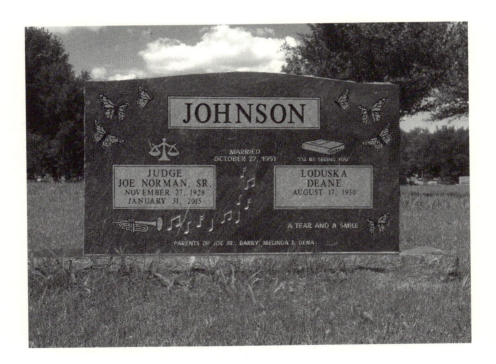

Special Letters

From Joe Johnson Jr. ("Jody")

I was privileged to be with my Dad last night when he passed away after an 11-year fight with Alzheimer's.

Dad was 86 and spent the last five years at a residential memory care facility in Waco. He has not been able to call us by name for eight years, but we always thought in his subconscious he knew us or at least knew that we were important in his life. Such was the case this weekend. When my brother and I arrived Friday night, my Dad blinked his eyes repeatedly when he heard our voices. We knew he recognized us. He was in a coma the entire time and was kept comfortable with hourly morphine. Our immediate family stayed with him until his death last night. The last couple of hours were difficult with a combination of lack of oxygen and gasping attempts at breathing. As death replaced life with a final breath, he opened his eyes widely for the first time since we had been there, as if looking at an incredible sight. A big grin spread across his face, then he was gone. In addition to our family, nurses and hospice personnel were present and saw the exact same gaze and expression that I saw. It was truly awesome.

Dad was the first person in his family to complete high school. He obtained a Bachelor's degree in Music and a Law degree from Baylor. He was an Army veteran, having served domestically and in France. Dad was a Justice of the Peace in McLennan County for 24 years, a District Judge for 16 years, and was a solo practitioner for 24 years. He was a hard-working, honest family man full of integrity. I am very proud of who he was and the impact he had on his family and community.

Dad's passion was music. He was an incredible trumpet player, touring the country with big bands in the late 1940's, fronting the Joe Johnson Orchestra for 15 years, and directing the Baylor Jazz Orchestra for many years as well. With Alzheimer's, the last memories you retain relate to your passion. This is why Dad was whistling, humming, and trying to sing until last Friday even though he had difficulty talking and could not recall any name or specific memory.

I actually had no intention of typing past line one of this email, but it feels good telling even a small part of Dad's story.

-Joe Johnson Jr. ("Jody")

From Tommy Riggs

Joe Is

(Written on January 31, 2015 after hearing of Joe's passing)

There are so many thoughts,
So many prayers, and so many notes.
We stop and think,
Paralyzed with ignorance
About what happens next,
Or about what has actually
already happened.

A life is lived, and that is truth
Within our accumulated understanding
Of life and living.
But then comes an event we call death,
And life, as we have defined it,
Ceases.
But then there is the ineffable truth
Of continued life and living.
We hardly begin to comprehend
Systems and galaxies and universes.

The smallness of our unknown existence
Is overwhelming.
This life and death and belief
In a future existence becomes reality.

Then we attribute it all to what we call God,
And are satisfied to define such a concept
As the source of all, from whom all comes,
And to whom all must return.

Our minds embrace life,
Our minds embrace death,
And our minds embrace life again
After death.

For it is with songs that we sing,
With music we play
And celebrate justice and law
As the way we do our defining
And thus do our freeing
Our minds and our consciousness
Of the vices and superfluities of life,
Thereby allowing the new life to enter,
The transition to take place,
And the celebration to begin in reality.
As souls progress, they carry with them
The concepts we mortals call love,
And hope, and faith, and trust
In the kinship of souls and spirits—
A kinship only briefly imagined and experienced
In our finite existence and finite kinship:
More complete and magnificent
To be experienced we know not how,
Not limited by time or space or other
Quantum attempts at understanding.

Joe is There,
Though we persist in trying to be exact as to location.
Joe is there now and forever,
Though we persist in trying to be exact as to how long and when.
Joe has been with us tangibly.
Joe is now with us intangibly.
Joe is recognizable,
Not with eyes, ears, face, body, and brain,
but as soul and spirit,
Which includes all we can imagine and more.

His smile is the warmth of the sunshine.
His being, his soul, his spirit,
Is one with God,
And one with us
Just as it always has been,
And just as it will always be.
Joe IS!
Halleujah!!!!!

Acknowledgments

To my children—Joe, Barry, Mindy, and Dena . . .

In 2003, we began a journey together. In the beginning of your Dad's memory-decline with Alzheimer's, I found myself in a dark forest with no compass. I know that, without meaning to, there were times I probably demanded more time, more visits, and more help from you to help me out of the forest. As a mother looking back, I know my expectations were unrealistic.

We all suffered in our own way watching this man who was our rock decline into the last stage of Alzheimer's. I never noticed anything but love and determination from each of you to be all you could be in the years of Joe's Alzheimer's decline. We were on a new planet without any idea of what was in store for us. I know that visiting Joe took its toll on each of you when you left to go back home. The body and mind was struck with an emotional tiredness that lasted more than a day. Going to see Joe after we moved him to Sodalis was never easy. I saw each of you take a step back at times, take a deep breath, then open the door with a smile on your face as if nothing had changed in our lives. You honored him. You watched his decline, and stood by his side until he took his last breath. I tried to be strong for all of you and Joe, but I didn't always achieve that goal. Joe lives on and watches over all of us.

Life after Joe's departure has affected us all. Speaking for myself and imagining how each of you feel is a new emptiness. It is a joy knowing Joe has escaped the debilitating effects of Alzheimer's, but it is difficult to remember what our lives were like before Alzheimer's. Your love and visitations to your Dad and to me were the greatest gifts to the man whose legacy you carry. Joe Johnson lives on in each of you: his mannerisms, his humor, his talents, his music, his love of mankind, his work ethic, and his love for his family and God.

We are never alone—God walks with us daily.

To Joe (Jody) . . .

I watched you, the oldest, take your place to comfort me and your Dad. I saw a new connection between the two of you—Joe, unable to express his feelings in words, and you, holding his hand to comfort him. A new kind of father-son connection in the pitfalls of Alzheimer's emerged. The son was in the role of father to his own father.

To Barry . . .

After reading your reflection in my book, *I'll Be Seeing You*, I realized that visiting with us was difficult. As difficult as it was, I was impressed by the ways you found to communicate with your Dad. You remembered every story he ever told you, and you became the storyteller, reminding Joe of his past. Humor and laughter encompassed every visit. You brought laughter to his declining life and never once did your pain show. Nothing is as good as a hearty laugh, and every visit from you was laughter.

To Mindy . . .

Daddy's little girl grew up fast. Your pain, camouflaged with gentleness, comforted Joe and me. I leaned on you and I depended on you for almost twelve years. I was never disappointed when I called for help. Your nickname from Joe was "Minner." Even during his Alzheimer's years, he seemed to know you. I know he was happy to see you even if he couldn't say your name. When I said "Minner," he knew who you were. You have a calming persona so much like your Dad.

To Dena . . .

Daddy's baby girl was stronger than I was. Dena, you have a knack just like your Dad to be frank and honest and in the same breath, gentle. Most of your visits were just the two of you, and I loved the one when you recorded him singing and took your boys by to see him. Dena, I don't know how Joe's disease affected you—I never saw sadness in you, only strength. Your name "Dena" was the one he called often while walking the halls at night. The workers said he did this often. When he knew you, he knew you as the baby of the family.

To Jackson and Eric (our grandsons) . . .

The two of you visited with your Boppa when he was in the end stage of life. Your reminiscing with him and your prayers were a great comfort to him and to me.

To The Good Folks At Sodalis . . .

We were blessed when I moved Joe to Sodalis in May of 2010. It was our home away from home. You became our family.

To Our Friends And Our Doctors . . .

I cherish each one of you. You were a comfort throughout this quagmire of Alzheimer's.

To Mike and Patti Paschall . . .

I first met you when you interviewed me for your book, *Till Death Do Us Part*. I knew immediately that we were kindred souls. You have been my rock, you have understood my grief, and you have been a comfort to me throughout my journey with Alzheimer's.

To Jonathan Hal Reynolds . . .

Jonathan helped with both of my books, but his talents didn't end when he finished. While reading my book *I'll Be Seeing You*, he made mental notes of Joe's and my first kiss, our anniversary, and Joe's last night at home. Jonathan sent me e-mails acknowledging these special days, as well as Thanksgiving, Christmas, and Joe's departure. A man of many talents and a man of deep feelings. We were remembered.

To J. R. Fleming . . .

J.R. is much more than an artist. She is in tune with my story. J.R. read my story and in essence told my story on the cover. I have been told by many people that the cover art of *I'll Be Seeing You* moved them to tears. That is the mark of a true Artist.

E-mails from Readers and Friends

Each semester for the past four years, I have spoken to a class called "Death and Dying" at Baylor University. My focus has been on the slow decline of the Alzheimer's patient and how I, as a wife and caregiver, traveled the bumpy road of fear while finding joy in the moment.

Following are two letters sent to the professor, Kay Tuel, after my visits to the class. -Deane

Professor Tuel,

I truly enjoyed your class this semester. Overall, my favorite part about your class was that you brought in guests who have experienced loss or are going through their own dying process. Of the guests, the one I appreciated most was Deane Johnson. Deane was the first person to really talk to me about Alzheimer's since the loss of my grandmother. Growing up, I remember witnessing my grandmother experience a sun down episode, and she started seeing people in the room with us. The last time I was able to see my grandma was the day she forgot who I was. I haven't allowed myself to go back to that memory until the day Mrs. Johnson came in and talked to us. When she was in the classroom, she asked if anyone had experienced a loss to Alzheimer's and I was the only person to raise my hand. When she pointed to me to give my story, I was at a loss of words. I felt like she knew that I was unable to talk about my loss, and she quickly took the attention off me and asked the class if they had ever lost a loved one. In that moment, I tried to make it look like I wasn't crying. That day was the first time I have ever cried in public that was not a funeral. I was sixteen years old and no one had warned me how different it would be to see my grandmother in that state. We sat with her until she passed, then went home and never discussed what had happened. I have never told this story to anyone because it is something we did not talk about as a family. Death is seen as a taboo discussion in my household, but in this class I learned it doesn't have to be that way. I feel like hearing the discussions about children and death is extremely important for health care professionals to be familiar with, because children are still a part of the family and they deserve to have their opinion heard and they need to feel open to talk about their grief. Deane's explanation of her husband was the first time I was able to hear another firsthand experience of Alzheimer's disease. I've read books about it, but being able to hear in person what someone has experienced is what we as future health care professionals need to hear. Without your class, I never would have called my Mom to talk to her about her mother's Alzheimer's disease. You were right . . . talking to someone about their loss won't upset them more, but it actually made my Mom happy to talk to me about her mother. We shared many memories that I never would have learned without your class. I'm sorry I couldn't say this in person, but thank you for teaching me so much. I truly feel as if I will be a better health-care professional because I was able to be a student in your class.

Hi Professor Tuel,

I graduated from Baylor this past May, and I took your class called "Death and Dying."

Right now, I am a first-year student at Emory University. We are in a class called "Growth Processes" and are talking a lot about Alzheimer's disease. I remember that we had a guest speaker in your class who talked about caring for her husband with Alzheimer's. If I remember correctly, I think she also wrote a book about it. I really think that my current professor would love to read it. Unfortunately, I cannot remember the guest speaker's name. If you wouldn't mind sending me her name or the name of her book, I think it would be a great resource for the class I am in.

Reply from Kay Tuel:

Our speaker was Deane Johnson. Her book is *I'll Be Seeing You*. I made a film of her that you may want to show your supervisor. It is only about 6 minutes, but it will set the scene for the book. On YouTube, look up "A Conversation on Grief: I'll Be Seeing You" with Deane Johnson.

Mrs. Johnson spoke again this past week. She said her husband is in a totally new stage now because he has regressed to the level of a two-year old. He can't feed himself, says "NO!" a lot, and can't hold any conversation. He walks in circles most of the day. So sad. I want to do a sequel to their story to tell about this phase of Alzheimer's. She is all for another film.

I received the following "remembrance emails" after Joe's passing and also from readers of I'll Be Seeing You. *-Deane*

As a Waco police detective, I often dropped into Judge Joe's J.P. office at the courthouse to get an arrest warrant. He would always see me coming and tell me in his booming voice to get my (blank) you know what in his office and talk to him. After some fun conversation, he would sign the legal paperwork I needed and I'd be on my way until the next time. The Waco and McLennan County community has lost a good guy and a great man. He will be missed. God bless his family and friends. —David K.

I am so sorry for your loss, but what a great man Judge Joe Johnson was! Twenty-four years ago, I asked Judge Johnson to swear me in as an attorney (out of my profound affection for him), and even found the oath that he was to use to make it official.

"There's an oath? I hope all the others took it," he said.

A great laugh was had by all.

I had the honor of practicing in front of him several times. I was always given a fair shake, and the hearing was always followed by a laugh. I hope you are comforted by the numerous lives he touched along the way. He was a true Gentleman. —Stan S.

Judge Johnson was a wonderful man. My ex-husband and I were one of the many couples that were married in his home in 1967. Judge Johnson also divorced us in 1991. After the divorce, he had a man-to-man talk with my ex. I also worked at the County. He was such a great Gentleman. My prayers to the family. –Mary Lou

Some of the most formative times of our high school days were spent at your home. I can hear your father's laugh right now—it was infectious. –Roy B. (to Jody)

Lu Ann contacted me recently and told me the sad news about your Dad passing away. He was a good guy and admired and respected by all. I have a lot of fond memories about your folks, but what I think of most is when we all used to sit around your den on Sunday afternoons watching the Cowboys play. I remember your Dad sitting in his chair by the back door with his legs propped up and making funny comments about the players, coaches, and the game. I specifically remember the game where the Cowboys came back against John Brodie and the 49ers, and I remember how we (including your Dad) were all jumping around and going nuts. Love To All, -Big O (to Jody)

I am so sorry for your loss. Joe was an important man in our lives at Sodalis, and I know even more in yours. From his music to his laughter, he will be truly missed. Knowing that he is no longer in pain doesn't make it better, but eases it a little. I love you and Joe as if y'all were blood. —Analicia (a nurse at Sodalis)

Mrs. Johnson,

My heart has been hurting for you this past week, and I've been thinking of you every day. I hope you've felt loved by many during this immensely difficult time.

I'm glad that you are still journaling, and being able to process your thoughts and feelings. You have gifted many with your words and shared experiences.

Let me know once you feel that you have finished documenting this part of your journey, and I will see if my schedule will allow me to work on any more projects at that time. In the meantime, write the truth, and know that I'm thinking of you.

    Much Love,
    Jonathan

Deane,

You are an awesome woman! I am so thankful for all those nights recording Joe's CD's with Joe and Kenny.

    -Dick Gimbel

Hello My Precious Deane,

Jackson texted Mike tonight sharing that your Joe is now with Jesus!

Also, I'm praying rest over you tonight and that peace will flood your heart knowing he is healed and whole again, united with his Mom and family and friends, and that there is no Alzheimer's in Heaven! Judge is playing in the jazz band on those golden streets!

Big, big hugs! I love you dearly!

    -Patti Paschall

Deane,

Thank you for writing your story about your journey. It was a good book to read—very helpful, sad, and happy all at the same time! Thank you again and I hope all is well with your family!

-Susan B. (from England)

Deane,

Do you know how much you are teaching all of us about what it means to love? Your very name speaks love.

-Jackie

If you would like to contact Deane,
please email her at: *deanejohnson@twc.com*

Visit Deane's website at:
www.deaneandjoe.com

Made in the USA
Middletown, DE
05 October 2022